Monique Doyle Spencer

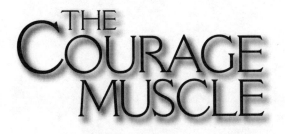

THE COURAGE MUSCLE

Here's to Sci For, for the
new ideas, solutions, potential,
collaboration and sheer genius!

This is a new idea too, for the
millions who struggle to _live_
with cancer.

Best,

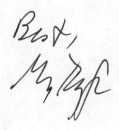

Monique Doyle Spencer

THE COURAGE MUSCLE

A CHICKEN'S GUIDE TO LIVING WTH
BREAST CANCER

CHANDLER HOUSE PRESS, INC.
Worcester, MA USA

ISBN 1-886284-74-1
Library of Congress Catalog Card Number 2004113488
First Edition
ABCDEFGHIJK

Published by
Chandler House Press, Inc.
335 Chandler Street
Worcester, MA 01602 USA

Design by Michele Italiano-Perla
Cover illustration by Paul Gilligan
Author photograph by Coffee Pond

Chandler House Press books are available at special discounts for bulk purchases. For information contact
Sales Department Chandler House Press – 508-756-7644 – 335 Chandler Street, Worcester, MA 01602,
USA or publishing@tatnuck.com

This book is designed for educational purposes only and should not be used in any other manner. This information is not intended to substitute for informed medical advice. You should not use this information to
diagnose or treat a health problem or disease without consulting with a qualified health care provider. A
consultation with your health care professional is the proper method to address your health concerns. You
are encouraged to consult your health care provider with any questions or concerns you may have regarding
your condition. Rapid advances in medicine may cause information contained herein to become outdated,
invalid or subject to debate. Accuracy cannot be guaranteed. Beth Israel Deaconess Medical Center assumes
no responsibility for the information presented in this book. Beth Israel Deaconess Medical Center does not
personally endorse any of the treatments, medications, articles, abstracts or products discussed in this book.

Preface

Paul F. Levy

There is not much to laugh at when you work in a downtown academic medical center. A tertiary hospital cares for the sickest of the sick, people with heart disease, strokes, diabetes, and, of course, cancer. We do the best we can to cure people, and, if that is not possible, to make them more comfortable. We try to do this with grace and respect, treating every patient as we would want our closest family members to be treated. Our doctors are skilled and the best in the world. Our nurses are compassionate, warm, and remarkably adept in handling a full range of medical problems. Our patient population is like a mini-United Nations, and we have translators who speak 32 languages to make sure they can be understood and can understand. We treat families, too, with social workers and case managers who do their best to help people through the anxiety and uncertainty of the hospital stay and, equally important, the recuperation afterwards. And finally, we offer palliative care for those who must spend the last days of their lives at our institution. In summary, our staff is seriously hard at work 24 hours a day, devoted to alleviating human suffering.

So, in the midst of all this serious business, Monique Doyle Spencer shows up with the story of her breast cancer treatment, *The Courage Muscle: A Chicken's Guide to Living With Breast Cancer*, and I start laughing. I worry. Am I being improperly irreverent? After all, my mother-in-law had breast cancer, and we barely smiled during her treatment, much less laughed. A good friend had breast cancer, and we all spent somber weeks figuratively and literally holding her hand. I was on the board of a breast cancer research institute with women who had had the disease, and I cannot ever remember laughing about the topic.

But here comes Monique, with her dry, incisive humor and she makes me laugh. Inspired by her I say, without thinking, "We will publish your book as a Beth Israel Deaconess Medical Center publication." In amazement she says: "But no publisher would accept it. They all think it is improper to make fun of this disease. Are you sure?" And I reply, "Absolutely."

Now, you need to understand that hospital presidents are trained not to make quick decisions. Instead, we carefully build consensus among a variety of strong-willed medical staff before committing to anything. As Monique left my office reality suddenly struck. What have I done? Here I am, with no training in medicine, social work, or the psychology of disease, having just committed our hospital to the publication of a book that experienced publishers have found offensive.

I faced a choice: I could forge ahead and get this book published or I could send the book to a group of our doctors, nurses, and social workers to get their review, taking the chance that they would find it unacceptable and then I would have to go back to Monique and renege on my promise….. A scary prospect – Not only is Monique a force of nature – she is smart and incisive and courageous. She faced the grim prospect of breast cancer, kept on smiling, and is intent on helping others do the same.

So, I did what any self-respecting American male would do. I signed the contract with the printing house and then told our doctors and nurses and social workers that we were publishing the book – their enthusiasm and support –see cover comments – has been "infectious." I want to thank them for their support of this book and for their commitment to making Beth Israel Deaconess the best.

You can help us change people's attitudes, too. Read the book and laugh. Then, tell people about the experience. Tell them to buy the book, too. The proceeds go to support Windows of Hope, a small shop near our oncology unit. The shops sells wigs, scarves, hats, and other items that are useful to people who are going through chemotherapy. More important, it has become a haven for men and women to share their stories and fears about cancer. Recently, too, with the publication of this book, it has become a place for people to laugh. We think that is good medicine.

PAUL F. LEVY

PRESIDENT AND CHIEF EXECUTIVE OFFICER
BETH ISRAEL DEACONESS MEDICAL CENTER
BOSTON, MA

Welcome

DEAR READER! Cancer has so many heroes, but I'm not one of them. When I was diagnosed with breast cancer, I knew in my heart that I would fail to meet any challenge ahead. I had seen cancer heroes and was sure that I lacked just about every quality you need to face this.

I therefore planned a treatment year of depression, whining and complaining, interrupted by long naps. Then, to my horror, I began to hear that a positive attitude helps you to beat cancer. No one knows why yet, and it's not foolproof. Plenty of whiners survive and plenty of strong, positive people don't. But overall, oncologists will tell you that your outlook will help your odds.

Oh, great. Just when I had the world's best excuse to drop out for a year, I'm supposed to have courage; just when I feel at my most afraid, I'm supposed to develop a positive attitude. How is a new cancer patient supposed to do any of that?

Do you feel the same way? Many of us do.

You're reading this because you or someone you love has cancer. I wrote this because somehow, in the early days of chemotherapy, something began to change. People were commenting on my positive attitude. I couldn't believe it, but it was starting to be true. I started to write down what I was doing, because I could see growth taking place and I wanted to share it with other patients and their families and friends.

As this attitude increased in me, treatment became easier to face. Not easy, still, but easier. I discovered that you don't actually have to do a whole lot to get started, because courage is a dormant muscle in all of us. Someday, we'll discover that it has its own place in the brain, and that most of the time it sleeps. But this muscle, like adrenaline, can spring into action for you when you need it most. It can happen quickly, or slowly, but *it happens for all of us.*

Now that you've been diagnosed, your courage muscle is already coming to life. I learned some simple steps to help it along. I hope that these can help strengthen your own courage muscle so that you can relax and watch it grow.

I wrote this while I was in treatment, either chemotherapy, surgery or radiation. I wanted it to be a real account of what happens, unsoftened by distant memory. I also wanted it to remind me that most of us – the vast majority – will survive cancer. It is a major challenge, yes, but not a death sentence. This reminder helped me to laugh at many things that happened, as I hope you will. Laughter, good loud laughter, is too much for your courage muscle to sleep through.

I don't know if you are at the beginning, middle or end of treatment. Standing here at the end, I can promise you that life can and does become wonderful and hopeful again. The more you are open to letting your courage muscle grow, the sooner that will happen.

I wish you well, and you know by now that when one cancer patient says that to another, even if we've never met, she means it.

MONIQUE DOYLE SPENCER

...But God, I'm a Chicken

DOES THIS SOUND LIKE YOU? A doctor is saying something to me but I'm still day-dreaming, as usual. I'm standing at Disney World. My 13-year old talked me into trying the Tower of Terror, that ride where they drop you 13 stories in an elevator shaft. I've handled it really well, I think. My teenager wants to wait to see those photos that Disney World takes at the scariest moment of every ride. Ours is ready now. There are about 20 people in it and I can't find myself at first.

Nineteen of the people are having a great time. They're looking straight into the camera, arms up like on a roller coaster, laughing and thinking what a great ride this is. The last person, me, is crying, hanging on for dear life, eyes squeezed so tightly shut that they've disappeared, screaming so much that the woman behind me is touching my shoulder and comforting me. "It's okay," she's saying, "it'll be over in a minute."

The doctor is now yammering in such a sweet, kind voice that I'm starting to think I must have something really bad. I can't have cancer, I think, because I know I can't handle it, because I'm a chicken, always have been, always will be.

During treatment I would often come across messages that made me laugh, gave me hope, or reminded me to look outside myself. I would write them down and stick them in my pocket or bag, then read through them when I felt like it. You'll find some too.

I've noticed that there are no chickens with cancer. The world has so many heroes, and in cancer treatment you hear about a lot of them. There's cyclist Lance Armstrong, who survived cancer that had spread to his brain and went on to win the Tour de France more than anyone ever has. There's Jockey Bob Champion, who went on to win the Grand National. His horse, Aldaniti, was a medical hero, too, and has a clinic named after him in England. Then you turn on the Olympics and begin to feel that everybody but you already has cancer and you can't even run down the street. Oh, God, back up a minute, even the horse wasn't a chicken.

Other people become living saints. She never complains! He is so patient and kind! She is so spiritual! He's become so prayerful! I have a sinking feeling that I am not going to do very well in this club of cancer patients.

You hear about cancer heroes from everyone around you. "My cousin didn't miss a day of work. My sister's husband left her, she still raised her seven children and she didn't miss a day of work. My uncle invented anti-gravity boots, my brother cured the common cold, my friend climbed Mount Everest." Sure, but did she miss any work?

I looked up cancer books online. I found 1,275 of them, many about people who fought incredible odds with valiant courage and found faith along the way. I didn't do any of those things, but I led a happy life through treatment, with plenty of laughter and joy along the way. I think I figured out how to live the rest of my life without being paralyzed by non-stop fear that cancer will come back.

I'm writing about it now because I was able to do this, one of the hardest achievements of my life, even though I am and remain a royal chicken. We chickens have to get through the challenges of life just like everyone else, but we don't think we can. We know we can't, we know we can't, we know we can't. If you are a fellow chicken, you know the feeling. But to be a chicken and survive is to know a kind of bravery that fills you down to your toes.

Right now, maybe you're reeling with shock from your diagnosis. Maybe you're terrified that it will kill you, or wishing it would so you wouldn't have to deal with treatment; maybe you feel scared not knowing what's going to happen, or scared that you do know what's going to happen and you bet it's not good.

Whatever you are, you're going to need some courage to face cancer, but most of us don't know where to find it. How does a chicken like you and me cross the months from diagnosis to survival?

Take a deep breath first. Remember *that most of us are going to survive cancer*; chances are that the odds are on your side. This is still going to be a big challenge, but so many of us will have a happy non-ending. Are the odds not in your favor? Then you're going to need to reach pretty deep to handle all of this, but you're going to have plenty of help.

Courage is closely related to the famous positive attitude you're going to hear so much about now that you have cancer. Everybody's going to tell you about it, how you *have* to have it, how it saved Uncle Harry, well he turned out not to have cancer at all, just gas, but whatever.

But some people, when they say that you must have a "positive attitude," mean this: "Please don't bother me with your feelings. I would rather not hear about cancer at all." You are almost guaranteed to feel this from someone at some point.

But people who *love* you say "positive attitude" because they want so much for you to survive this and they've heard that your attitude can help. Of course, if they read in a magazine tonight that worms and peat moss might cure you, bet on seeing worms and peat moss in your oat bran tomorrow morning. But these people have got it right. What they mean by positive attitude is important.

A positive attitude is just this: your fundamental belief that life goes on with you or without you, so it may as well be with you. You want to survive and believe that you will. How it acts out in you is your choice. If it is a quiet and serene conviction that you will survive, fine. If it means you start dotting your i's with hearts and smiley faces, fine. You are posting poetry everywhere? Buying lots of angels? Or kicking ass and swearing a lot and laughing yourself

silly at inappropriate moments? All fine. Your life will go on, it is worth living, you're in good shape.

The challenge? If you are reading this without a cancer diagnosis, these
sound like greeting card sentiments, don't they? But during cancer treatment,
it's a little different. If your reaction to treatment is hard, *you still have to keep
going back*. It helps a lot if you want to survive and believe that you will. What
seems like something from an
embroidered pillow now becomes a
lifeline later.

This plan starts with your
diagnosis, with a few tips on how to
get your mind around it. Like all big
problems, you'll take this one apart
into all of its smaller pieces first.

Next we try to anticipate
some challenges ahead and plan
how to meet them, in order to free
your mind for the more important
task of healing. The plan works on
finding your strengths and figuring
out how to be yourself, because the
stress of being someone else all the
time distracts your mind from healing. This is all part of deciding how
you and (for now) only you want things to go.

THE 30-SECOND POSITIVE ATTITUDE

The famous positive attitude
you hear about is really this:
a fundamental belief
that you will survive ...
and that you want to.

How that shows in you
is up to your personality:
You can be walking sunshine.
You can be serenely prayerful.
You can eat Bitch Bar for breakfast
and wash your tamoxifen down
with a shot of whiskey.
You know your life will go on?
It's worth living?

Then you're in good shape.
You are just fine.

Next is building your courage muscle and setting a few life-giving goals
— the foundation of the plan. I've added some topics that I found useful after
that: how to deal with "helpful" people; how doctors and patients could talk
with each other; a detour for a personal experience with faith or lack there-
of, or "what I found when I got in the foxhole where they put all the atheists."

Some tips on treatment come next, followed by housework, which I have no business writing about, and trying to get used to your new body. Then on to the future, which you aren't even thinking about yet, but which yawns ahead a bit at the end of treatment.

At the end of the book you'll find a research plan, a list of resources, a notebook to use and some thanks to the people who helped me along this stupid, godawful, inspiring and rewarding road.

Sorry, Wrong Number!
The Diagnosis

YOU'VE BEEN GIVEN THE INITIAL NEWS. I could start this chapter with a poetic description of my own shock and share the depth of my feelings with you, including how my husband and I held each other and sang each other folk songs or something. But I have something more important to say, which is this: Call your dentist right away and schedule a cleaning. You won't be able to go for months if you're having chemotherapy, and the resulting dental work is a good bit worse than cancer in my opinion, so do yourself a favor and go now.

That important stuff is now taken care of. Anyway, you've been diagnosed. You don't know much about it, because you have more tests to have first. Before you go to the step of learning more about your individual cancer, you'll be letting your diagnosis sink in, which is going to take awhile. One good way to receive your diagnosis is with prayer and grace. I hoped that would work for me, but discovered that another good way is, well, with anger and swearing. Someday scientists will discover why this helps, but until then, I just believe. I take it on faith.

"What does not kill me, makes me stronger." *

So many people said this to me that I looked it up. It was first said by Friedrich Nietzsche, the philosopher and atheist, who, as you might imagine, then ...
* Died at the age of 56.

Many people say that, emotionally, this period is the lowest point of cancer. That's true. You really are going to feel brighter, you really are going to survive this, life really will be wonderful again, but you won't believe that for a while. Try writing Psalm 30 on a note card and sticking it in your wallet: "Weeping may linger for the night, but Joy comes in the morning." If I were a blasphemous person, I would call this the "manic-depressive psalm," but good thing I'm not. I find it very comforting and hope that it will help you.

You might then make a detour to wonder what you did to cause this cancer. This isn't too useful, since nobody, not even a smoker, plans to get cancer, but for some reason we need to wonder what we did. Do yourself a favor and wonder this out loud so you'll hear what it sounds like. Then you'll stop.

After you finish swearing you jump to "I'm dying." You'll wonder what it means to get your affairs in order, because you've never been able to do that when you thought you would live forever, and it seems as if the one good thing about dying young would be that you could at least leave that mess behind for someone else to deal with. Congressman Joe Moakley, dying of cancer, said he "didn't know how anyone dies without three months notice." In the meantime, you have questions, serious questions, about your prognosis. We all find a different way to express that question, like whether we should buy green bananas or not. Mine was: Should I bother catching up on those thank-you notes from my wedding 16 years ago, or can I finally, finally, finally forget about them?

You discover one good thing: you could plan your own funeral, pick all the songs you like, you could start going to services now so that the Priest/Rabbi/Imam/Minister (or P.R.I.M.) will know you and be able to say good things about you. You'll have time to say quotable things to your best friend and remind her of all the wonderful qualities you have that might be mentioned in a eulogy. You can pick the epitaph for your grave marker.

My favorite: "I *told* you I was sick."

Still, you probably feel you're dying. All kidding aside for a moment. If you have kids, that feeling could kill you if the cancer doesn't. This grief is profound, the deepest you've ever felt. The tears you'll cry now will give you no relief or solace and you'll ache from the heart. You'll feel a despair that will be a heavy physical burden, so deeply does it sink you. Your dreams will take you to the darkest places in your soul and you'll fear going to sleep, except that being awake is so, so much worse.

Then you start to realize that you are grieving as if *the kids* are dying, not you. Try repeating that a few times. You feel that way just because you might not see them grow up. You are grieving for all of the things you might not see.

Then you realize, with relief, that *they are going to grow up with you or without you.* You think of all of the wonderful people you've met who lost their parents and survived very well, even with all the pain of losing a mother. You can just grieve for yourself now, which is so much easier. Sounds simple, but it takes awhile to get to that point. In the meantime it's really bad, the most painful thing I've ever felt. I would stand over my sleeping kids and pray and pray and pray, and then pray some more, followed by more prayer, and then, for something new, I would start to pray.

Note to my teenager: not that I stood over your sleeping form, because I would never, ever enter your room without your express permission, so I stayed in my room and just thought about you. Yep. And I never once stroked your hair or kissed you while you were sleeping, since – and let's be clear about this - I was not in your room. Which, by the way, is a godawful mess, and there are new life forms growing in that orange juice glass from last summer, and don't tell me you need more clothes with that mountain of jeans in there.

Your kids will ask you point blank if you're going to die. My answer was that there was no reason to think I would. I would take my medicine and do everything I had to do to get better. We all believe that I'll be fine. If anything ever changes, I'll tell you right away. So you can relax, honey, and do you have any questions?

My kids were 14 and 9 when I was diagnosed, so my information is for that age group. With any age group, half the task is what you communicate with your attitude, so I kept mine strong, low key and positive.

That's my view of it, but my kids say that I kept my attitude weak, martyred and negative. They imitate me lying in bed asking for ice cream in a whiny, self-pitying voice, as if I were crossing the desert and begging for water.

Anyway, your job is to talk carefully and seriously but without making a big deal of it. Cry or rant to your poor friends, not your kids.

This talk won't be the last conversation you'll have. You'll need to reassure them along the way. Just keep your attitude low key around them. No fake enthusiasm, no high drama, just matter of fact speech. And remember that they are always noticing. They'll notice an increase in answering machine messages from your doctor, for example. Inform them about each milestone along the way, simply, straightforwardly, positively. They're going to learn a lot from you and about you now.

If you have teenagers, you are not expected to get through this without ever toying with them or trying to make them feel guilty. Everything in moderation, you know.

Most of all, when kids are afraid you're going to die, they mostly just want to know who is going to take care of them. I told my kids who would take care of them and that was enough. "Cool!" they said. "We *love* them!"

Your next step is to find out how bad this news is. Most cancers are assigned a stage, which tells you how advanced your cancer is. In breast cancer, there are four stages, plus a stage 0 that is very early or small and sometimes not considered to be cancer, but try convincing your fears of that.

If you are anything less than Stage 4, which most of us are, do yourself a favor and be happy and relieved and overjoyed for a moment. Yes, you're going to have a challenging time, but your chances are just so good.

There are plenty of Stage 4s who also do very well – it's just that I am limiting my ramblings to anything up to Stage 3, because that's what I have. I don't know how it feels to be Stage 4; one of the themes of this book is that if you don't really know anything about someone else's feelings then first be quiet; then listen; then shut up again. I'm shutting up.

THESE ARE THE BREAST CANCER STAGES.

STAGE 0

In many places you won't see this stage mentioned, because it is a very, very early cancer or even a pre-cancerous condition. It is tiny and has not spread anywhere.

STAGE I

The tumor is small and it's local. It has not spread to the lymph nodes. The tumor size at the largest part is 2 centimeters (cm) or less. Two cm is as big as this line: _____.

STAGE 2

The tumor measures up to 5 cm, which is about two inches; there is no involvement of the skin or ribcage; up to three lymph nodes may be involved. Or, Stage 2 may mean a larger tumor, bigger than two inches, but with no spread to the lymph nodes, skin or ribcage.

A lymph node is like a turkey baster, taking liquid from one place and sending it to another. The liquid is lymph, which is a clear fluid, from a word meaning spring water. Lymph goes all over your body, doing a few jobs, such as carrying antibodies to fight infection.

Lymph nodes are little organs that keep it all moving. You have lots of lymph nodes under your arm, in your neck, around your chest and other places. Your surgeon will want to remove nodes that have cancer in them. You can live without some of your lymph nodes, but they make the body's job easier.

STAGE 3

The tumor is bigger than 5 cm (about two inches), with spread to the lymph nodes. Or, the tumor is smaller than 5 cm but there are four or more nodes involved. Or, you have any tumor that involves the skin or ribcage.

STAGE 4

The cancer has spread from the breast to other parts of the body, such as bones or organs. This is metastatic cancer.

Measurements are always given in centimeters because scientists don't have time to read the paper so they don't know that everybody else gave up on the metric system right after the Carter administration. Anyway, you'll likely have tests to find out what stage you are, and then you'll work with your team to figure out the best treatment. They'll be looking at a few factors beyond your stage, such as how aggressive your cancer appears to be, how old you are, if your tumor likes estrogen or not. No book or website can tell you what treatment is best for you. For some cancers, there are just a few options, for others there are many.

A note on your stage. I was stunned to find that I was Stage 3. I had gone for my mammogram every year and it was fine. How could I be this far along? I learned that not all cancers show up on a mammogram. A small percentage resemble the density of breast tissue and are not visible. So, I had a tumor that was huge but could not be felt and was still invisible on the film. This isn't an excuse to skip your mammogram, nor is it a BITTER TIRADE that I've gone EVERY YEAR and it DID ME NO DAMN GOOD. No. It's encouragement to do self-exams and go to your annual physical and have an exam. MRIs and ultrasound may be used, who knows when, but I suspect that even then we'll still have to do self-exams.

The other message is to take lumps seriously. I woke up one morning feeling like someone had put a big egg in my breast. You could actually see it. It would have been easy to assume that a sudden big lump is just a cyst, but fortunately my doctor didn't. While it's true that most lumps are just lumps, you still have to check them.

TWO DOCTORS, THREE OPINIONS?

Now, just when you desperately want to simplify everything in your life, everyone will be telling you to get more and more opinions. I think that is true if you have a serious diagnosis, but not all cancers are rocket science, so you'll have to decide if you want to get third and fourth opinions or not. I vote yes for seconds, but your situation will guide you from there. The more serious or complicated your case, the more opinions you should seek, the more research you will want to do. If it's really serious, you'll want to become an expert.

And guess what? You'll still be confused. This isn't strep throat you've got. If it were, you'd only get one answer, of course, which would be comforting. But this isn't a game of Jeopardy where one person knows the answer and you just have to figure out which doctor is Alex Trebek. It can be complicated, and if you put the time in now to find yourself a team you like and trust at this point, it will pay off later. That's also true if your cancer is in an early stage, because there can be plenty of debate about what to do and how aggressively to treat your tumor.

You want to understand the reasons for your course of treatment. If your second opinion agrees with your first, it's awfully nice. It gives you a bit of extra confidence in your treatment and your team. There's a chance, however, that it will be different, in which case you may want a third opinion. The reality is that you can get many professional opinions and still have no idea which way to go. In that case, you're going to be making a decision that is as well informed as possible. You're going to feel confused along the way and there's no way around that, but it will help you feel better if you learn more.

If you're like me you're going to be overwhelmed and maybe even bored by the number of websites, books and services out there, so at the end of the book you'll find a two part research plan. You pick how much you want to know and then gather information from the books, phone numbers and web sites listed. You can choose any level of information you want as you look around on the web, ranging from sites that say, "This is a boob. You have two.

Oops! Let's count them again." to sites that are about "the contralateral superficial inferior epigastric artery flap," which is a real article in which I correctly understood exactly two words: "the" and "flap."

A great comprehensive and helpful website to start with is www.Komen.org. When I was diagnosed in 2001, my second favorite discovery was a website operated by the Department of Defense. I don't know why the Department of Defense is so very interested in breasts but I'm sure it has something to do with national security or maybe just protecting the great American breast. I can't find this site anymore so breast interest might change with each administration.

One bit of advice: with all research you do, be sure you are looking at information on your specific type of cancer. Cancers are all different with different treatments.

YOU AND YOUR LUCKY STARS

Right after you call everyone you know and make them panic, then cry your head off, then go to the dentist, here's your next step. Look honestly at your life and answer this question: Is this the worst thing that ever happened to you?

If it is, take a moment, go outside and thank your lucky stars. You've had an easy-ish life. Throw this book if that makes you mad to hear. The good news: this challenge is going to retrain you in ways that will make you strong for anything else to come along.

If it's not the worst thing that's ever happened to you, you already know you're going to be okay. But maybe with your luck you should quit buying lottery tickets.

I did do some research, but that wasn't the most helpful part of my learning stage. The most helpful thing was to interview people who have been in similar circumstances. A lot of people will offer to put you in touch with a cancer survivor, way too many for you to call. I had to tell people that I really enjoyed talking with survivors but I was a little worn out.

The helpful calls? People who are the same stage. If you are Stage 1, find someone Stage 1. The last thing you need is a Stage 4 wondering why the hell you think you have problems. If you are a 4, the last thing you need is a Stage 3 telling you how helpful her Pilates classes were and how you must go. For once in your life, stick to your own kind, one of your own kind.

Talking to people who have been through treatment will give you the range of individual responses people experience. I talked with people who threw up with every treatment, but most people don't. Most people reported fatigue, but everybody had it differently. While I wanted certainty, to know everything that would happen to me and when, everyone helped me to realize that I could survive without it. It's just like any other life experience: the only way through it is through it. You're not going to research your way to knowing every minute that is to come. But learning from other people is always good; just keep the wide range of responses in mind so that you're open to your own path. And only interview people you like.

WHERE TO GO?

Part of your task is also choosing where you will be treated. Ask your doctor, ask any doctor you've ever met, ask anyone what they think is the best place in your area.

Then add in some practical matters. If you live near a city, you have a few choices, so consider how convenient one site is over another. Sounds crazy now, but when you are going for radiation every day you'll sure wish they were closer and had better parking. I hope you were warned that this book is shallow and superficial, but to me parking is one of the deepest issues of life, and if that makes me shallow, well, it's not easy to remain a superficial person when you have cancer, but I'm trying my best.

Looking at how people choose their doctors, I've heard a lot of people talk about having an adversarial relationship with them. They have to keep pushing and prodding and demanding. Sometimes that is the patient's own personality at work, and if you gave them a different doctor it would take *all* the fun out of having cancer.

I need to trust the people who are treating me, so if I felt that I had to be my own doctor every step of the way, I would switch to someone else. You don't need to love them, they don't have to be your friends, but you have to be able to trust them at a basic level. The golden rule of trusting a doctor? Don't trust one who says "Trust me." If they can't or won't answer questions, run as quickly as your IV bag will allow. To a hopefully nearby and reasonably priced parking space.

My oncologist was a good match for me. He would explain everything and he would give me the pros and the cons, at the level of information I needed. He treated my husband the same way. There were no surprises from start to finish. By his manner he made me feel that my progress was important to him, which gave me confidence. He kept on top of my interactions with other specialists and always knew what was going on. He gave me certainty when he could but was always direct with me. I didn't know when I met him that he is very well known for all of those traits. By the end of treatment, I had learned that the human quality of my team was incredibly life-giving. I didn't know how important that was at the beginning.

Not every doctor is wonderful. Neither is every hospital. But if you keep asking everyone you know, you'll quickly arrive at the best decision for your area.

Stepping on the soapbox for a moment, there are two conditions that are very tough combined with cancer: rural locations and poverty. You'll find resources elsewhere in the book for addressing transportation problems and money woes. But if I could say one thing on this subject, it would be: if you yourself, or anyone you know, is living in poverty or living in a rural area or both, it really is a matter of life to have your physicals on time. Even more than most people, you need early detection. Early detection can mean that you have surgery, perhaps with radiation and hormone therapy, for example. But late detection can mean that you can add months of chemotherapy on top of that, and that's going to be pretty tough under your circumstances.

Very often, the earlier your cancer is found, the cheaper and shorter the treatment. Please see Chapter 17 for more.

Besides: the big problem with cancer is not that it will kill you, but that it *won't*. For most of us, early detection is not about avoiding death — it's about avoiding as much treatment as possible. So next time you're tempted to put off an exam, take a moment to realize that avoidance can therefore be a deeply selfish thing to do to your family. I'm sure you know people who sound quite proud of their doctor-avoidance. "Haven't seen a doctor in five years," says the proud man with the family history of heart disease, cancer, diabetes and bad judgment. He could be tested now and be fine, but instead his family will have to carry him through months of treatment.

BREAST SURGERY

This section is here, early in the book, because many people have to make decisions about surgery very early in their treatment. Breast cancer has quite a few possibilities.

There may be two surgeons involved, a breast surgeon and a plastic surgeon if you are having reconstruction. The breast surgeon does the cancer removing. The plastic doc remakes the breast if you choose to.

Your breast surgeon will first look at how extensive the cancer surgery needs to be. A mastectomy, in which the breast is removed? A lumpectomy, in which part of it is? If you have any concern about this, be sure to get a second opinion. I felt confident that mastectomy was the way to go. You want to feel confident in your surgery, too. Unfortunately, when it comes to surgery, your doctor's total confidence isn't a good indicator. Surgeons are famous for confidence. You know the Latin on your surgeon's diploma? It means "Often Wrong, Never in Doubt." I was lucky to have human surgeons who were not at all arrogant. But not everybody is so lucky, so I'm encouraging you to get a second opinion about your surgery.

When I met my breast surgeon, I had heard non-stop praise about her. Women of all different stripes just love her and I was amazed by the fervor of what I heard. To my delight, everything I heard was true. I thought she would float in on a cloud with a ray of sunbeams and the Ave Maria going full blast from a choir of angels. And so she did, except the choir was from Chippendales.

I was offered the option of having half of my chemo first, before surgery. Typically surgery comes first, but they are sometimes offering this option because it reduces the tumor. For some women who do it this way, this is the difference between a lumpectomy and a mastectomy. Nobody expected that to happen in my case, but I picked this option because it would push my surgery to the summer, and childcare is easier for me in the summer. (Because you can just leave the kids out in the backyard all night.)

This option had a nice extra benefit for me: since I still had my tumor, I could actually see and feel the difference in the size of it with each chemo treatment. Mentally, this meant that the chemo was working and I liked that. This isn't something so important that I would use it to make a decision; it was just kind of nice.

The decisions about reconstruction are completely different. The good news is that you don't have to decide all at once. You can have your cancer surgery and do the reconstruction later. You'll hear a lot of debate about this among surgeons and oncologists, and even psychologists. Some people feel that you shouldn't make a decision about reconstruction while you are dealing with the emotions of breast cancer. Others say your emotional life will be easier if you have reconstruction right away. Some people say that the reconstruction should wait until after all of your other treatment is finished, because radiation may mess up your reconstructed breast and because complications from surgery could delay treatment. Some hospitals may not even give you the choice of doing everything at once because of these concerns.

I received many different opinions on this timing question. I finally decided to do everything at once, from mastectomy through reconstruction, with a side order of breast reduction. I had no medical reason for the decision. I was simply way, way too chicken to face surgery more than once. I did have some complications, which did delay some treatment. My reconstruction surgeon made sure I understood all of the potential risks before agreeing to this timing, so I went into it fully informed. To my amazement, nobody said, "I told you so."

Whatever you do, nipple reconstruction will come later. It's not done at the same time as reconstruction, because your breasts need time to settle before this final step. Nipple reconstruction involves a skin graft for the center, and tattooing for the circle around it.

Www.breastcancer.org has some good discussions about this timing issue, but it's one that you want to look at with your whole team. For all of the major decisions, in fact, you want to touch base with the different specialists who are caring for you.

After surgery I swore off bras forever, so the first day of cold weather was pretty funny. One breast has a nipple, the other doesn't, so the colder it got beneath my sweater, the more I looked like my breasts were winking. I'm not sure I want to give up this little novelty, but in a few months I'll probably get tired of it and opt for the nipple.

Your surgeon will also be looking at the best *way* to reconstruct your breast if you want to. The options include implants or reconstruction using your own tissue from the back or abdomen. The back is an easier recovery; the abdomen tends to look better and gives you a free tummy tuck at the same time. My abdomen couldn't be used. More about the back below.

Most women can have reconstruction if they want to. Just don't let anyone push you one way or the other. I've seen women be pressured by their friends to refuse reconstruction on some vague political grounds; I've seen women pressured to have it by their boyfriends on sexual grounds; I've seen mothers who had radical mastectomies want their daughters to do or not do the same.

Also, you are about to be initiated into the amazing world of reconstruction surgery, which is the medical term for "plastic surgery that your insurance company pays for." How amazing is it? Remember, *my new breast was made out of a muscle from my back.* They take a muscle from your back or abdomen, sneak it quietly to your chest, and make a breast out of it. Now, these surgeons have done so many of these that they don't remember how unbelievably insane this sounds to the new-comer. But I can guess the story of this particular innova-tion.

First, it involved alco-hol, mixed with a group of medical students. These med-ical students were male, and I mean that in the nicest possi-ble way, not to suggest that a group of men put together with alcohol would necessari-ly always think of something stupid to do, and by this I also don't mean my husband or my brothers or any gentlemen reading this book. Anyhow, medical students have the kind of status that would get them really great dates if they had time, which they don't.

WHY ARE YOU SO WORRIED WHEN THEY "GOT IT IN TIME?"

Are you a nice early Stage with no lymph involvement, so everybody just wants you to "move on?" Remember that you may know that your cancer is a nice early one, but your inner chicken does not. You'll eventually feel glad that you have a nice Stage, but it's going to take awhile for you to feel that way. Give it time. And tell that cousin who needs twelve people to take her to her mammogram but who keeps saying you should not be worried, to, well, you know.

Why do some people insist that you should not be worried? Read the Circle Theory chapter for more.

So one night, a group of them who happened to be men were "studying." One of them, who was destined to live through his twenties without time for a sin-gle date, wondered idly yet scientifically what you could make a spare breast out of if you had to.

They started with stuff around the room, like stitching inflated rubber gloves to themselves, which historians now believe is the origin of implants.

But then they drank a little more, and a little more, and then somebody said "Hey! I know!" and the first one who passed out woke up in the morning with a rather large breast and a missing back muscle. Sadly, this ended his career, because, as scientists have observed, if you give a man his own breast he will stay home for the rest of his life to play with it.

I'm very, very sure this is what happened because no other explanation makes any sense whatsoever. The history of breast reconstruction surgery makes me think of the pride we can all feel when someday there is a class of *female* medical students sitting around wondering idly yet scientifically what they could make a spare you-know-what out of. Fortunately, girls learn very early in life that you should always, always be the very last one to fall asleep at slumber parties, so nothing will come of it.

Anyway, whatever mix of chemotherapy or radiation you have could be complicated, or it could be pretty straightforward without a whole lot of choices.

It's often the surgery that involves some decisions for many of us. You'll have some puzzling days in which you'll try to decide what to do about your own surgery. Your doctor will help but will most likely not make the decision for you. Explore the options and the risks, and then make a choice. Drive yourself crazy if you want to, but an informed choice is the best you can do, because there are always unpredictable events. You can't predict the outcome with 100 percent certainty, so all you can do is *make a choice based on the best information.* For example, I had some tissue that didn't do very well after surgery, which meant a whole round of nursing care that I didn't expect. If I had known for sure that that would happen, would I still have done all my surgery at once? Sure, because you couldn't have *convinced* me in advance that it *would* happen.

And also because one of the nurses I then met taught me to use the word "fooker," a term of endearment for your husband, for example, that in Ireland rhymes with "looker." It is used in many phrases, such as "That fooker's late again. I am going to kick that fooker to the curb." Or: "I'm through with that fooker."

I wouldn't have missed that bit of knowledge for the world.

SUMMARY SO FAR:

Now you know your stage and where you'll be treated. The next important step is to let your fears relax a bit and then lay down some basic plans. We'll begin to get your mind around this.

She looked as though there were nothing on earth
she would not look at like that, and really she was afraid of so many things.
—Ernest Hemingway, from The Sun Also Rises

Getting To Know Your Inner Chicken

HOW POORLY PREPARED do you feel for cancer? I keep looking for people who were as scared as I was because it makes me feel better. Have you found out yet just how loud your inner chicken is? Mine was screaming – so loudly that it created a good time to explore fear and try to understand it.

We have two kinds of fear in us, both woven into how we react to life. One is the powerful but rational reaction to an event. This is adult fear, the kind you feel when something is really threatening.

The other is more complicated, because it is fear rooted in the many years you spent as a child, totally unable to control your surroundings. It is not rational and it makes your heart pound. Fear of abandonment, fear of spiders, haunted houses, Keith Richards, those centipede lashes on the old Tammy Faye. The fear that towers over you in your childhood nightmares.

This childhood fear is so strong in us that it made Freud utter his only known words that were not about sex. Freud says that this insecurity creates belief in God; in our helpless childhood, we create God. Even God says, hmmm, this childhood fear is so strong that maybe Freud has a point there.

It is useful to learn to separate these two kinds of fear, because you have both wandering around in your mind, and they are holding hands. It's hard to tell the difference. Fear of cancer is an adult, rational reaction. You can manage this fear, overcome it, live with it, get over it.

The child fear? *Fear* of nausea, for example. Fear of *needles*. Ain't nothing you can do about that except close your eyes really, really tight and whimper. This is the fear that freezes you in your tracks. There are probably therapies for fear of needles, I don't know, because I fear those fear therapies.

I've always loved horses so I decided to learn to ride. Bear with me, this is relevant.

I loved it, rode twice a week for a long time, but I spent every single minute of it afraid. Before you dismiss me as even more terminally chicken than you are, please listen a minute: I was riding twice every week *without ever actually being any good at it*. I fell often. I paid many visits to emergency rooms. I was thrown, bucked, run away with, bitten and stepped on.

So I had every good rational reason to be afraid of horseback riding, based on the direct evidence that it was bad for me. But I could love it anyway, scary or not, and still choose to do it.

Horses weigh about half a ton, and could think of ways to kill you if they felt like it or weren't quite so, well, stupid. Guinea pigs, on the other hand, weigh a couple of ounces, could fit in your pocket, and live to please. When the kids were old enough for pets, we thought guinea pigs would be a good place to start. I was able to live with my fear of big thundering horses, but the cute little rat pigs? Nope. It took me three years before I could pick one up, and even then I was screaming "Oh my God, oh my God, oh my God, oh my God" until I put it down. How about beetles? Centipedes? I need to go lie down now before my heart jumps out of my chest.

The pigs give me that visceral child fear. There is nothing I can do about that but some deep breathing and screaming. Remember Franklin Roosevelt saying that we have nothing to fear but fear itself? Now I understand that. He had obviously been frightened by a few guinea pigs in his life, or maybe by that mother of his, and lived to tell the tale. He knew fear when it came knocking.

The point is that this child fear is hard to live with. You couldn't live with it everyday if you tried. As a chicken, you may be afraid that you'll be spending your treatment life and post-treatment life feeling like *that*.

Your adult fear, however, is a different animal, and thank God it's a horse and not a guinea pig. You can reason with it, train it, tame it. You will still be afraid, but it will be a fear you can live with, not at all like your heart pounding fear of (fill in the blank).

The more you can unclutter your mind by separating these two fear cousins -- adult fear and child fear -- the freer you will be to understand the adult fears you do have and overcome them or live with them. You can let your child fear flutter away. This frees you to listen to your adult fears, to have a good long chat with them and about them, and to live with them while you're in treatment. After all, they're going to be your close companions throughout your life, so you may as well get acquainted.

Getting Started: Basic planning for your treatment year

MY FRIEND TIM TOLD ME THIS JOKE: "How do you make God laugh? Just tell him your plans."

Even though that's true, we're still going to develop a plan. It's a big part of freeing your mind to do the important jobs it has to do. Without a plan, your mind is going to keep itself busy with details all of the time, and you won't have the mental room to find strength. You're no doubt going to need to be flexible during treatment, but it's still a good idea to have an over-all plan. It starts with the tangible issues and then you can develop some emotional thoughts that will be your guiding philosophy.

It's a whole lot easier to do it if you can feel a little calm about the sheer practical arrangements of life. So first, nail down your physical treatment plan. It will likely be some combination of surgery, chemotherapy and/or radiation. My schedule was three months of chemo, followed by surgery (a mastectomy and breast reconstruction, with a breast reduction on the non-cancer side), then a little physical therapy, a second three months of chemotherapy, followed by six weeks of radiation and then a plan to take tamoxifen for five years.

Yours may be the same or different. If you are being treated for prostate cancer, chances are good that you'll be able to skip the breast reconstruction surgery, unless your surgeon has some kind of bet going with the other surgeons.

Write down the general schedule that you and your doctors come up with. Jot down some thoughts about each stage, and what your biggest practical concerns are. See which ones you can plan in advance to alleviate. Everyone's life is different, so your concerns may be your work, insurance, transportation, childcare, your marriage, dating, money, your faith, your meals, even your appearance.

I had reduced my work schedule greatly to handle a previous crisis, so I was in good shape there. Many people obviously continue to work, but you still can count on some sick days. After your first round of chemotherapy you'll have a good sense of how the physical things go, except that most of us do get more fatigued with each treatment.

You won't be able to plan for everything now, but try to get a good start. Keep in mind that chemotherapy is an amazingly individual thing. I've seen weak little things waltz through it, and strong big things struggle. This is not one of those things that everyone says is "individual" but we all really know isn't – like how our kids' soccer abilities are just "individual," not "really bad." With chemotherapy, it really is individual. You can't know how it's going to affect you until you've done it. The only constant is that they have a lot of stuff today to help you with comfort, so ask.

Back to the plan. For me there would be childcare needs so I began planning for that. Insurance? Rights? Better find out now. (Did you know that a 1998 federal law requires your insurance company to pay for matching breasts after mastectomy?) Marriage? I love mine, but my plan was still to keep paying attention to it. Transportation? If it's going to be a problem, talk with your hospital, which will know about services to help out. My faith? Well, there's a chapter about that later on, but don't read it if blasphemy gives you the willies. Money? Again, talk with the hospital because they are likely to know about resources in your area. You can also try cancercare.org on the Internet for resources on financial help, because cancer can be a challenge if you are already having financial troubles. This site lists a lot of them and gives advice on finding local help. Cancercare.org also gives you resources for finding transportation.

Work? Check out www.cancerandcareers.org. It ranges from employee rights to cosmetic help and is worth a look. Also check out the CIS book mentioned in the Cancer Research Plan.

Dating? Hmmm. I don't know. In movies this is a really great time to date because the guys seem to love falling for women with cancer. I don't have the experience in real life to know, but if it were me I would at least try keeping it up.

Meals? I was the luckiest person in the world. I had married a really good cook, first of all. But then, our close friend Jane Morgenstern, along with a teacher at school (and friend), Janyce Lee, organized 30 families to give us a month of dinners after my surgery. It was a godsend.

Do you live in a neighborhood like that, or belong to a church, synagogue, temple, ashram or mosque that might help when you really need it? Don't say no to help. I had absolutely no idea that there were that many wonderful people in my community but they came out in force and helped us. I felt like I was living in "It's a Wonderful Life" and it still makes me a little teary.

SUMMARY SO FAR:

Write down a general schedule for the treatment year in the Notebook section. Identify areas that worry you — Insurance? Transportation? Childcare? Make any plans you can to handle those areas, plan around them, or rely on someone else to do them.

On to appearance. In my personal plan I was not going to care about how I looked. God laughed at that plan, so I ended up spending $75 on eyeliner alone. As a little aside here, just wait until you walk through that old department store cosmetic department with no hair and no eyelashes. Nobody, but nobody, will be offering to help you now. They will be all of a sudden so distracted by any old thing they can think of that somehow they miss you. Note to self: consider shaving head for Christmas shopping season. In fairness to good people, thanks to the wonderful woman at the Bobbi Brown counter.

Stop now. You've done everything you need to do before you start treatment. Your job will be to start treatment now and start to get your mind around it and how it's going to fit into your life. When you feel a little bit of calm about the physical and practical arrangements, on to the emotional part.

CHECK YOUR REAR VIEW MIRROR BEFORE ACCELERATING

You may feel overwhelmed now by the practical arrangements, or you may feel better. For me this was a good time for a healthy dose of perspective. If you look back over your life, is this honestly the worst thing that ever happened to you? If it is, take a moment, go outside and thank your lucky stars. You've had an easy-ish life. This challenge is going to re-train you in ways that will make you strong for anything else to come along.

If it's not the worst thing that's ever happened to you, you already know you're going to be okay.

I've learned lessons about perspective from so many people who have problems much worse than mine as well as from people who are more like me. I also learned that perspective has two angles. The first is the life view, knowing that you are truly fortunate. The second angle of perspective is how you view specific problems. My favorite perspective lesson of that type was one I got from the diaper man. My little one had gotten some tummy bug, and I was up to my nose in orange poo. It had been a long week and I was almost ready to trade my little angel in for a somewhat drier species.

The diaper man came to the door. I told him that I needed a lot more this week because of the tummy bug. He smiled and patted the baby on the head. "That's my little money maker," he said. "Keep up that good work, Punkin'."

When I was in treatment, Martha Stewart's troubles were in the distant future, so I could write about her without kicking someone who is down. A friend told me that she can't watch Martha Stewart. It depresses her and reminds her of her inadequacies as a homemaker. I LOVE Martha! I told her. I have watched her show several times, and each time it was like a vacation from all my worries. Why? Because *there's* a woman who is a little nuts. If I'm feeling a little on the crazy side, a little Martha is a mental health break. Aaaah, I think, I'm doing *fine*. Compared to Martha, I am the picture of perfect sanity.

I could watch Martha all day, but it's time to get the frozen hot dogs out for dinner and then go on to emotional challenges.

SUMMARY SO FAR
Think about who you are. What works best for you in coping?
Practice choosing how you feel about small events.

Who Are You?

RIGHT NOW YOU MAY NOT HAVE ANY IDEA who you are, but you'll find that cancer makes you find out. It's one of the great benefits of cancer if you're open to it.

Why ask who you are? The idea here is simple: Your body has a lot of work to do, and it needs your mind to help it out. The best way for this to happen is for your mind to be at its best, and that happens when you are yourself and when you are operating from strength.

This chapter is about choosing your own way of handling your treatment. You will be trying to find a way to handle some combination of surgery, chemotherapy and radiation. I believe strongly now that if you choose your own emotional path through this maze, it will just plain be easier for you.

Fans, for the past two weeks you have been reading
about a bad break I got.
Yet today, I consider myself the luckiest man
on the face of the Earth.
—Lou Gehrig

I chose this quote for this chapter because it is the single best
example I've ever heard of a person who chooses to be joyful
against all odds. It was my favorite inspiration, also because Gehrig
worked on youth projects in New York after retiring from baseball.

We'll start off with some preliminary thoughts: who are you? What guiding ideas will work best for you? Then you'll set a few general goals. And then you'll check in with yourself once a week and see how it's working.

First, spend some time getting to know your own treatment personality. These ideas about your treatment personality will be sketchy in the beginning, but try it anyway.

Ask people who know you well for some observations on things you do really well, especially in coping with crises. (I stole this approach from a wonderful sister-in-law.) Then see if you can find some connections between your strengths and the challenges of treatment. Are you a serious person, low-key in your manner? Fine. You'll be able to learn to reduce the stresses of treatment and you'll find comfort in information. Other people may be volcanoes of grief, with everything falling apart, but not you.

Do you handle a crisis better when everyone else falls apart? Fine, because you'll have plenty of opportunity. Are you funny and loud? Fine. You'll release a few endorphins to help you battle stress. Do you take pride in your appearance? Fine. You'll find that you have a new face to put to its best advantage. You'll have fun with jewelry, make-up, hats, scarves and you'll look great too. Old joke for prostate patients: it's even more exciting for women.

My statement was this: *I am going to go to bed for a year and whine the whole time.*

That's who I thought I was and I told the medical team they would have no trouble reaching me, because there is a phone next to my bed. Don't call during naptime, I said, which will be from dawn to dusk, followed closely by bedtime. I said it out loud to many people. I'm still surprised to find out that I'm someone else entirely, and that may happen to you too. But let's start at least with some idea of who you are.

One of the things you'll learn soon is how your own personality wants information. Many people find it comforting to begin treatment armed with every piece of information they can learn. You may be one of them and do lots of research. They look at all treatment options. They know everything there is to know about conventional medicine, alternative medicine, mind-body connections. They seek information hungrily and are eager to talk with anyone who might have helpful knowledge. They make careful and informed decisions about their care and where to seek it. They know every web site there is. They might even begin a nutrition and exercise program. All of that is what we should do.

My own preparation, however, consisted of drinking a pitcher of Sangria and smoking a cigar. My thorough background check on my oncologist consisted of thinking that I liked him. Of course, I felt that I had the luxury of making decisions this way since I was going to the Beth Israel Deaconess, which was supposed to be one of the best hospitals.

Looking back, how did I know that? Because I saw it on The Simpsons. Marge breaks a bone. The ambulance pulls up, with a sign on its front saying "Springfield City Public Hospital" or something like that. Homer says, "No, no, no, you can't take her there – take her to the best place in town! Money is no object!" So they change the sign, and now the ambulance is going to "Beth Israel." At this point Homer panics and says "D'oh! It doesn't have to be *that* good!" They settle on a lesser place, but I don't have to. Fictional or not, Beth Israel Deaconess it is.

That was my initial reaction, but then I did get second opinions and I did do research. After the whirlwind of diagnosis, tests, and preparation, I was supposed to be ready to start chemotherapy. All I knew was that I didn't know anything. The team repeated everything three times, but only one fact had stuck in my head. The only fact was this: "Before each treatment, Mrs. Spencer, we will weigh you."

I laughed. A hollow, empty laugh. Of course you will, I thought, because cancer and chemotherapy just aren't enough. You need to weigh me too. On this day, I start to learn how I will handle this kind of thing. "You're welcome to weigh me," I say, "as long as I can weigh you." Everyone laughs and I feel better.

They think I am kidding until I drag a doctor by the hair to the scale, screaming. This feels good, I think, and I jot it down as a "coping strategy."

Some people find great comfort in information and knowledge, and that can be very important. This taught me one of my first lessons about cancer treatment, that we all do it a little differently with the same outcome. I didn't find cancer very interesting as a subject and I never loved research.

Last night, though, I spent time online researching cancer and all of the terms on my pathology report that I couldn't remember what they meant. I looked around at all kinds of web sites, which is a really big mistake at midnight when it's cold in the house and your feet are freezing. Do you know what I mean? My spirits got lower and lower until by 2:00 I knew I would be dead by morning. As far as I can tell this didn't happen as it turns out.

I remember having a blood test and a friend asking me what my numbers were. I'm thinking "lottery ticket," and if my numbers came up I'm not sharing with you. No, no, your hema-something numbers! she says. I had no idea. In the future, I always asked for my numbers so I could answer the questions. These weren't cancer numbers, which at this point don't reliably exist for breast cancer. These were post-chemo blood tests. I think they do it to make sure that they are making you sick enough with the treatment. And, "knowing my numbers" proved to be more helpful than I thought, because I learned that I "have great numbers." I liked telling people my numbers and having them tell me that my numbers are great. It meant that my bone marrow was terrific, which must be good, maybe from eating that bone marrow appetizer all those years ago. See the section on "Diarrhea" to learn more.

I never could answer most of the questions people asked me. But I learned not to judge people who become experts on cancer, just as I hoped they wouldn't judge me. After all, they are more helpful to their friends and family over a lifetime than I am. They are a big help to people who are newly diagnosed or are in treatment.

Whether you become an expert or not, *this doesn't mean that you stop paying attention. You are a chicken, not an idiot.* Know any and all of the numbers that will help you track your progress, because they can inspire you. *You have to pay attention to all drugs and treatments that are given to you and understand them clearly. Please stop and re-read this paragraph.* Why? I remember a nurse changing my IV pump as she started the chemo. I asked her why, and she explained that "this stuff eats through plastic." So, this stuff eats through plastic, said my chemo buddy, which can last for 1000 years in a landfill, but you're going to put it in my veins?

This ain't aspirin they're giving you, and you need to be paying attention *to everything that is happening during treatment and make sure that everything is triple checked.*

At each treatment I thought of Betsy Lehman, a health writer for the Boston Globe who died of a chemotherapy overdose in another hospital. I never met her, but as I watch the nurses check and re-check everything together, I wonder how many deaths she prevented.

In general, while I kept my technical cancer knowledge at a low level, I eventually learned a lot about the people who were treating me. For me, that was more comforting and helpful. Different strokes.

FINDING CANCER BOOKS TO MATCH WHO YOU ARE

It may seem odd to start talking about books in the Who Are You stage. But people are going to start giving them to you, or you're going to start looking for them. This can be very helpful, but it can also be not very helpful, so I want to stress here that not all books are going to be good for you.

I did have moments of wanting to do some reading. Usually this happened when someone gave me a book about cancer and then asked me fifteen times if I had read it. (Note to self: remember not to do this to people anymore.)

These books were torture. They have subjects like How To Maintain Your Loving Sex Life While You Have Cancer. Looking Your Best While You Have Cancer. Keeping Your Skin Beautiful While You Have Cancer. Fitness and Diet While You Have Cancer. Communicating Effectively With Your

Teenager While You Have Cancer. And of course, How Not To Miss a Day Of Work While You Have Cancer.

These books should be called: "Here Is A List of Things You've Never Done For Two Days Straight In Your Whole Life But Will Be Expected to Do While You Have Cancer."

Luckily, I stopped trying to improve myself years ago, when I read my first Pregnancy Book. The chapters were: How To Maintain Your Loving Sex Life While You Are Pregnant. Looking Your Best While You Are Pregnant. Keeping Your Skin Beautiful While You Are Pregnant. Fitness and Diet While You Are Pregnant.

You get the idea.

No one else can judge which books are a good match for you. When you have the energy, go to the library or the bookstore and browse until you find what you need for now. You'll make a few trips like this, because your needs will change as you progress.

I can tell you what books were a good match for me. I liked survivor stories, like Lance Armstrong's *It's Not About the Bike*. My reconstruction surgeon recommended it and I loved it. Keep in mind that Armstrong had a very aggressive and very advanced form of cancer, which most of us don't, so the treatment he describes is much more challenging than what most of us have. I loved this book, which believe it or not is an easy read. You'll hear lots of good things about the book; my favorite was watching him grow up.

I also liked a practical book, *Woman to Woman: A Handbook for Women Newly Diagnosed With Breast Cancer* by Hester Hill Schnipper and Joan Feinberg Berns. It's short and it covers a lot of basics, including some tips that are very helpful. In a completely different category, try the *Survivor's Guide to Breast Cancer: a Couple's Story of Faith, Hope and Love* by Robert C. Fore, Rorie E. Fore and Nancy W. Dickey. The title made me barf at first, but it's an interesting format. It reads as a journal kept by both husband and wife and I liked that.

There are many hundreds of books. There are practical guides, advocacy books, inspirational survivor stories, alternative treatment guides. As you know by now, I didn't want to spend a lot of time becoming an expert. I tended to look for lots of information packed in one place, like *Woman to Woman* and also *Bosom Buddies: Lessons and Laughter on Breast Health and Cancer* by Rosie O'Donnell, Tracy Chutorian Semler and Deborah Axelrod. You'll find people who don't like the humor in it, but even if you don't there's lots of information. Humor about cancer is a funny thing; it's a lot like ethnic humor. If you're not Italian, your Italian jokes are not funny even if people laugh. I say that since Rosie O'Donnell's mother died of breast cancer, Rosie qualifies and can say whatever she wants.

I can't say that I've read every word of very many cancer books. You may want to immerse yourself in them, especially if your cancer is complicated. In any case, more books are listed at the end of the book in the Cancer Research Plan section.

The single best thing I read was an article by Stephen Jay Gould called *The Median Isn't the Message*, published in his book *Bully for Brontosaurus*. I read this after learning that the five-year survival rate for Stage 3 breast cancer is about 50 percent. At the time, that sounded pretty bad to me, until I read Gould's article, which has the best explanation of cancer statistics and what they don't mean. (Gould lived twenty years longer than he was supposed to.)

I know, I know, all you Stage 4s, 50 percent sounds great, but I didn't know that yet. Gould's article was sent to me by my dear uncle Paul. I read it many times and it was very comforting. I kept it on my nightstand reading pile for months.

WAKE-UP CALL

Anyway, time for the first chemo treatment. Michael and I go to the Oncology Reception area, and God sends me my first miracle.

My miracle will sound strange. On that day, a beautiful one outside, the waiting area was filled with a miserable collection of human beings. Rude, mean, nasty to the staff. On no other day have the people been this way. Usually everyone is feeling that we're all in the same boat, and everyone is pretty gracious. But on this Wednesday, I never saw a higher percentage of unhappy, unpleasant people anyplace in my life. After a few minutes of looking around, I turned to Michael. "I don't care how many days I have left. I am not spending a single minute behaving like *that*."

I go to the treatment area. Next to my little station is a couple a little older than we are. The woman is coifed in a turban, receiving her dose. Good Morning, she says, and smiles. Her husband smiles. We smile back. Life feels better. This is before I threw up.

I had learned a big lesson – that how I feel on most days, even with cancer, is a choice, and it's a choice that only I can make. In one corner, here are people with cancer who are miserable. In the other corner, a woman with cancer, same disease, same treatment, who is gracious and warm.

But — if you are chronically down with a bone crushing systemic depression, that's not what I mean. I've been there too, and the only way out is therapy, medication, prayer, exercise and time. No amount of "choosing your feelings" is going to get you out.

No, I mean "I feel this way because of *fill-in-the-blank*." The cancer I have. The driver who cuts me off. The woman at the PTO who always looks me up and down as if she can't believe I would buy these clothes. The guy at work who calls me Honey. The relative who spreads bad news. In the week before Election Day, I hate my husband every time we talk and I cannot believe I married him. Very depressing.

These things that make you feel one way or another aren't always small. How you feel when your mother dies. When you have a miscarriage after waiting forever. When your child is seriously ill. When year in and year out, every piece of news in your life is bad. When you have cancer.

I had never handled any of these events with any courage at all. I didn't even have the courage to talk with people about them, because I usually hated what people would say. "It's a blessing," they say so often. Your mother dies too young, you lose a baby. I never could see the blessings in these things. I would just retreat as far as possible. I still do that sometimes.

I decided to practice making all of my feelings into choices. I started in the hospital's garage. I end up, as usual, behind a 200-year-old driver in a gigantic car who cannot make a single turn. My blood begins to boil. I take a deep breath and decide to choose how I react. Well, I think, someday I will be that age, and I hope that the young person behind me will be patient. And, his car hasn't got a single dent, where mine has, well, "experience."

This didn't work at all. I was still totally irritated and sped around him. I will try again tomorrow, I think, when a friend is driving me in.

God, naturally, made sure I learned my lesson. My friend turned into a 300-year-old-driver with a gigantic car who cannot make a single turn, and I hoped that the young driver behind me was patient.

My second miracle came on my second day of radiation. The machines were broken, everybody was delayed, and I received the same wake up call I received at the beginning of chemotherapy. The patients, all but two, were ballistic, all in meltdown mode. Storming out, raising their voices, lots of "I will not be kept waiting."

Then I notice the young woman across from me. She is not a patient, but her husband is. He is in a wheelchair and is visibly ill. He is going to be admitted unexpectedly because they have found a blood clot. She is on her cell phone making arrangements for the kids, like I am, because of the delays. Except that she is talking to her teenager, who doesn't have her house key, about how she is going to get in the house … to get her *insulin*. Throughout these calls, this woman does not raise her voice.

The other person not in meltdown mode is me. I have exactly 25 people coming for dinner. I have to get my teenager all over town for medical appointments. My husband is out of town, the babysitter's car broke down, you name it, I don't have time for this three-hour delay. But how the heck am I going to get upset when this woman isn't?

The other piece that made this fun was that it was Halloween. The staff, in a moment of frivolity that must be the hallmark of radiation profes-sionals, decided to dress up for the holiday. And so, as they face a waiting room filled with hostile, angry, nasty cancer patients, they must do so wear-ing costumes. You can see how easy it was for me to choose not to get too upset. "Sorry for the delay," says Yoda, I think. "We appreciate your patience," says a man festively arrayed in red tights.

It was just like that first day in oncology. I could choose how I would react, so I did. The staff was not doing this intentionally, or incompetently, so it just didn't piss me off. Plus, I got to feel morally superior to all of the peo-ple who were melting down. I jot this down as yet another coping strategy.

I would have some not so bright moments in the year to come. Maybe there are cancer patients who sail through without a glum minute, but not me. As focused as I was on how I was going to handle this disease and its treatment, I still had moments of fury and despair. In other moments I want-ed my mom to come over, put me to bed, make me some hot chocolate and read me a story. Luckily, my husband and kids and friends would do it instead.

So, I started my treatment year. I had the physical plan started and I was ready to think about the emotional part more clearly. I had learned the first big lesson, that you choose how you respond to things. But at this point, I still know that whatever happens, I will no doubt handle it badly.

Seven things to think about when your mind wants to dwell on cancer:
Love of life. Love of children.
Love of husbands, wives, partners, family and friends.
Prayer. Friendship. Fear of death. Laughter.

These things, good Lord, that we pray forgive us Thy grace to labor for.
—Thomas More

The Courage Muscle Step-By-Step Plan

I HAVE ALWAYS WANTED to handle things well — even with courage. I am Woman, hear me roar. Instead, I am Scooby-Doo, watch me run. Or, if you're old enough, I am Snagglepuss, see me exit stage left.

When I was diagnosed I knew I was looking at a challenging period of about a year. It might be more or less for you, but I think we all have the same choice regardless of how long it's going to take: am I going to write off this year? Which was, by far, my first choice.

Unfortunately, I decided that a year is just too long to blow off, too much of my allotted time to waste. Could I really whimper for a year? Could I go to bed and complain? To be honest, with no children in my life I might have done just that. After all, remember the Beach Boy composer Brian Wilson - he went to bed for three years, didn't he? And he didn't have cancer, he was just in a really, really bad mood and had taken advantage of a few too many recreational options, I think. Why can't I do that?

Then I looked at my kids, and knew that they couldn't afford for me to drop out for a year. And I would love to set a positive example for them – so they will see how a crisis can be handled, and so they won't be too worried.

Here's what I decided: I don't know how many years I have left, so I can't afford to waste one of them.

But how on earth would I do it? Cluck, cluck?

You have the same choice to make. I won't blame you, and nobody else should, if you decide to go to bed and whine. If you decide that you can't waste a year, more or less, well, hooray. I've been through nine steps so far on my little journey. They didn't happen in any organized sequence, and I bounced around between steps as I groped my way along. But I hope they help you.

DO SOME HOMEWORK ON HEROES.

I began to think about heroes, just plain courageous people. John F. Kennedy, when asked as a young man how he became a war hero, said: "It was involuntary. They sank my boat." When I asked my mother how she had taken care of five children with the mumps when she had the mumps herself, she said: "I had to. I didn't have a choice." "And sit up straight."

I began asking people whose courage I admire just where they found their strength. The answer was so often the same, lots of different versions of "It was involuntary."

This was when I began to understand that courage is a latent quality in every one of us. This muscle comes alive for you when you need it most — quickly, or slowly, but it happens for all of us.

How else can we explain that every crisis in human history has brought forth heroes? Ordinary people save lives, fight fires, survive devastating loss. A fire happens in a building and there will be heroes, as there will be in floods, tornadoes, famines, wars.

It helps to learn about other heroes in all walks of life, so try to interview a few for yourself.

What strengthens that muscle? Love of life. Love of children. Love of husbands, wives, partners, family and friends. Prayer. Friendship. Fear of death. Laughter. The more you think about those seven things, the stronger the courage muscle seems to grow. I don't know why, but it does. Try writing these on another card for your wallet. For you, there will be other thoughts that help, too, so add those to your card.

In the meantime, your homework will probably teach you what it taught me: cancer is involuntary, and it's going to make that courage muscle wake up and start strengthening.

REMEMBER THAT YOU CAN DO A THING OR TWO.

Do you ever surprise yourself by handling something better than you thought you would? Don't you love that feeling? When I awoke from surgery, everyone said how great I was doing. I knew in my heart that I was going to handle surgery badly. I had never handled it well in my life, and I was terrified. But that night and the next day, the surgeons, who had put in a 10-hour session on this operation, made me feel wonderful. My husband, the nurses, everyone told me they thought I was doing great. I was inspired. I walked up and down that hall as fast as I could.

Not actually fast enough, given that I peed on the floor, for which I apologize to the patient in Room 5 who walked out of his room in his socks. I have learned that one of the many advantages of cancer is that no man is able to confront a 5 foot 10 mostly bald woman on morphine and demand to know why his socks are wet. Something about the way I look seems to say that you won't like the answer. I jot this down as another "coping strategy."

And then … the evil twins came on board, a resident and a nurse, who both relentlessly goaded me — I was ready to go home, they said, tomorrow. This is 24 hours after surgery, and I'm lying there thinking that if I go home I'm going to die. Why didn't I just tell them off? Looking back, I had had consistently positive experiences at the hospital and I was in no shape to realize how wrong these two were. I thought they must be right. It always amazes me when people have the presence of mind to handle a situation forcefully while they are still in it. I don't. For most of us, this is just a reminder that it's so helpful to have someone with you to help you notice and deal with everything.

Anyway, these two keep it up, and I become more and more depressed. I must be a weakling – even a chicken, I think, because they think I should be ready to go home, and I'm not. I spend a sleepless night, feeling terrible about myself, feeling very nervous about going home, feeling the kind of fear that only comes in the middle of the night when you can't sleep. I keep repeating Vince Lombardi's line to myself, "fatigue makes cowards of us all, fatigue makes cowards of us all." That usually helps, but it didn't now.

I wasn't okay again until I could see my real doctors. And rat on those two. By then I was calling them Dr. and Mrs. Harry Paratestes. If that didn't make you laugh please read it again.

Looking back, I had learned a lesson about expectations. We humans – which does not, even generously, count the resident and the nurse – *like to exceed expectations*. I felt great when the surgeons made me feel that I was doing better than expected. But when the bar was raised so high that I could never reach it, I just felt worse and worse. I didn't feel as compelled to walk or to do any of the things that were good for me. That post-surgery breathing exerciser, for example, that looks like it could be a bong, if you are old enough to know what I mean, but is disappointingly empty.

In having cancer, you've stepped into the biggest expectations game there is. Little is known about the mind and its role in survival, but anybody in medical care will tell you that attitude counts. So nobody wants to give you negative expectations for fear that they will somehow *cause* problems for you. "Oh, you'll feel fine in chemo, you'll feel fine." "You'll have minor discomfort after this procedure." This is so destructive, because it gives you expectations you can't possibly meet, let alone exceed.

This is one thing I loved about my oncologist. He gave me straight information about everything. I was never, not once, unpleasantly surprised. His manner said "I want you to do really well, and I know you can. It could be easy, but it may not be, *and either way we're going to be with you every step.*" I wish everybody did that, because if attitude really does count, they could work miracles.

I wish doctors and nurses never, ever said "this won't hurt" when it's going to. It defeats our attitudes before we get a chance to make them positive. "I must be a weakling," we think, "because that doesn't bother anybody but me."

Years ago I had laparoscopic surgery that I found quite painful when I was recovering. No pain medication is needed, the doctor told me. I really suffered for several days. Two years later, I ran into the same doctor again, because she was there to discharge me after I had given birth. She asked me if I was having contractions when I nursed. Sure, I said. Without being asked, she gave me a prescription for 20 major painkillers.

You guessed it – by then she had had a baby. She had learned a thing or two about pain. She could not give me enough painkillers. I wanted to slap her. "This won't hurt a bit," I would coo. "No pain medication will be necessary."

I had read in one otherwise good book that the tattooing they do before radiation is "painless." I would agree wholeheartedly, as long as you are under a rhinoceros at the time and the needle comes nowhere near you, because the rhinoceros is under an elephant. Otherwise, you should be entitled to one "youch" per tattoo. You should be allowed to look angrily at the tattooist and have your brow soothed by an attendant.

Okay, it only hurts for a nanosecond, but still. And sadly, the tattoo is delivered by a radiation therapist, where I had counted on a back room and a scary guy in one of those sleeveless T-shirts.

If this expectations business sounds like a good fit for you, talk with your treatment team if they set the bar too high. Ask them to be straight with you at all times. Tell them that you'll bring the positive attitude if they'll bring the good information.

Exceeding a few expectations — your own — is a good way to start exercising your courage muscle. Choosing some goals is a good place to start. Your first goal is to go to chemotherapy, or whichever part of this is scaring you the most. Just go. That is a big enough goal to begin with, and anyone who doesn't think so just hasn't done it.

As you become accustomed to the routines of treatment, your goals will be broader. But remember that goals should be goals, not mountains – something a little out of your reach, something that needs striving, like walking in the hall. But to expect a person to do something that you yourself couldn't do if you were covered in Fatima medals is cruel. And it just doesn't work. Having goals while you have cancer is great, inspiring, life-giving and important, but they have to be goals that are yours and that are based on reality. I used to believe a wonderful saying that if you aim for the moon, you may strike an eagle, but if you aim for the eagle, you'll strike only a rock. I believed that for a long time until I realized how much time and energy it uses. Get really good at striking that eagle seems a lot smarter to me now.

SUMMARY SO FAR You've done a few things before, and you can do this. Don't believe that it's going to be easy, but believe that you can do it.

It's involuntary.

FINDING YOUR OVERALL GOALS AND WAKING UP YOUR COURAGE MUSCLE.

I love the expression "You can't make a strong sailor on a smooth sea." You know how true that is – that we all need a little friction or challenge to make us stronger. You're not on a smooth sea now, and won't be for a while, so you may as well become a strong sailor.

To me, the best way to be the strong sailor at the end of the day, and not the one hanging over the rail for dear life and begging for the wind not to bring it right back to you, is to set a few goals.

Why set goals? Because even a cancer patient – especially a cancer patient – needs to be striving most of the time. *Striving is life-giving. Striving reminds you that you have a long way to go until your life ends.*

If you are one of those overachievers who always make the rest of us look so bad, start with an important first step: Set your overall goals for "most days." There are days that are better off just plain written off, but it is true that many days can be as great as you want them to be.

THESE WERE MY GOALS:

ON MOST DAYS, I WILL LOOK FOR SOMETHING TO REMIND ME HOW WONDERFUL LIFE CAN BE AND HOW MUCH I HAVE TO LIVE FOR.

Does that sound like a cliché? I used to call it one, before cancer. But there are times in cancer treatment when the future doesn't look worth the effort, just like in everyday life. Do you ever have those moments? Things look so dark that you don't feel you can take another step. Life could go on just as well without you. What, you say, you never have those moments? Well, count your lucky stars again. The rest of us have to get busy when it's dark, and find a flashlight.

The one reminder that worked for me every single time was the sound of kids laughing. Even better was the sound of *me* laughing and the sound of my kids making me laugh, my favorite of all. Write down what will remind you. I posted mine on the inside front door of my house so I would see it when I left.

ON MOST DAYS, I WILL ASK MY BODY TO DO A LITTLE MORE THAN IT WANTS TO.

Everyone you know is going to tell you about this study that chemo patients feel less fatigue if they exercise. I kept waiting and hoping for the study showing that chocolate does the same thing, but while I was waiting I decided to try the exercise. I was in terrible shape.

I started with a slow walk down my driveway, and my driveway is very short. On the next day I walked to the house next door, the next day the house after that, and so on. I was lucky to have lots of encouragement from the neighborhood. Ruth Rubin would clap as I walked by and would leave encouraging notes in my mailbox. "Unbeatable you," she would write, and I started to believe her. By the time I was done with chemotherapy I could walk fast for 30 minutes every day and I felt great. But I will never say, "Oh, If I can do it anyone can, so it must be easy!" It isn't at all. If you want to try it, check out Covert Bailey's book *Fit or Fat*. But start with baby steps, and talk to your doctor first.

Physical achievement of any kind makes you feel good. I started doing basic free weights for the first time in years, and it felt fabulous. I loved going to the store to buy new weightlifting gloves with my bald head. Was I a cancer patient or a bald weightlifter in a circus? Who could tell?

ON MOST DAYS, I WILL DO ONE SMALL THING FOR SOMEONE ELSE.

This might be calling someone that I knew needed help, or dropping something off for a shelter, or taking the time to listen carefully. This helped me a lot, given that I started this whole thing as a royally selfish person. I would cringe guiltily whenever my nurse would say that "women are givers who put themselves last, and you have to learn to take care of yourself while you're in treatment." I finally confessed to them that I hadn't put myself last once in my life, except maybe if I was on line to do something unpleasant, like be spanked, then I put myself last.

ON MOST DAYS, I WILL DO SOMETHING TO CHALLENGE MY BRAIN.

Some days, this was just a crossword puzzle, some days it was learning a new subject. I became interested in geology and had fun trying to understand it. I did this because there can be a little fogginess from cancer treatment. As my friend said – I was getting so forgetful that "pretty soon I'd be able to hide my own Easter eggs." I started to love this concept – imagine the benefits. Oh, Look! Someone made dinner! You could read a favorite book over and over and not even know it - what a surprise ending! See *The Crying Game* over and over! So, I thought it would help to exercise my mind, and that it would help me to think positively, too. I'm sure that this helped me avoid that chemo fogginess, which some people even call "chemo brain." I'm sure that this helped me avoid that chemo fogginess, which some people even call "chemo brain."

Damn.

ON MOST DAYS, I WILL THINK ABOUT MY FAMILY AND FRIENDS AND NOT JUST ME.

When I was first diagnosed, my oncologist brother-in-law told me that cancer, emotionally, can be harder on spouses and family than on the patient. That sounded nuts to me, but he was right. The patient can occupy his mind with treatments, schedules, appointments, and on and on and on. The spouse just worries and tries not to show it too much.

The world gushes in to help the patient, while the spouse is expected to be coping. It's like being a bridegroom or a new parent – important, but not exactly the focus of attention. The younger your children, the harder life is going to be for partners. They are going to have more days of feeling and being on their own. It's going to wear them out and scare the beans out of them.

So, anything you can do is important. I thought it was helpful to make jokes about my husband's prospects as a dating single man if I didn't make it. "Look on the bright side," I would say. "This time around you've got a job and a nice car!" That's not the kind of "help" I mean. I mean doing something for each person in the family that you know *they* will love. On a bad day, this might be just *saying* something they will love.

Today, as I near the end of radiation, we've had the first snowfall. It is one of my favorite moments in life and I went out in my nightgown to catch a few flakes. It is usually my job to shovel, so I got dressed and zipped back outside. I wondered why my husband was already there. I cleaned off the car, started to shovel and made it down half a sidewalk. It was with a big thud in my heart that I realized I couldn't do it. That's why Michael was there. It was a heavy, wet snow, and between the mastectomy and the fatigue, my arms and shoulders were not up to the job.

Michael knew it well before I went out. I thought about how often he has finished a job for me since diagnosis. I hadn't noticed just how often it happens. It was one of those deep romantic and spiritual moments so I threw a few wet snowballs at him and went back inside.

I decided that I could at least do something nice for him. I made him an actual cooked breakfast, not what I usually serve, which is vitamins, half a newspaper and a diet soda. At least, that's what I serve ever since my daughter told her pre-school teacher that she had had M&M's and root beer for breakfast, for which there was a perfectly good explanation but anyway I've obviously improved the bill of fare quite a bit and reduced sugar to boot. I also gave my husband all three Sunday papers, each unopened, which is one of those gifts above rubies if you ask me.

You may be someone who cooks breakfast for your husband or wife every weekend, but my excuse is that everything my husband likes makes me gag: omelets with bizarre cheeses that smell exactly like public bathrooms in hot climates; oatmeal, which I thought you give up when you get your first job; and coffee, mined at the La Brea Tar Pits. So I decided to make him coffee with this breakfast, which I have not done for Michael since 1980, because it's just too hard. You have to check the weather reports in Sumatra to make sure that the beans are picked at the peak of flavor, or something like that. The beans must be ground just before you use them, according to Michael, or you may as well not drink coffee at all. I searched among his bean collection and chose one. I got out the grinder, which Michael spent a year researching before buying. Unfortunately, I did not bother to get out the grinder cover, which turned out to be important.

I performed the various incantations and ablutions and started the grinder. It's a strong little thing for its size, which I learned when it sprayed me with ground coffee with quite remarkable force.

It was now deep in every pore. My skin was brown from head to toe, amazingly brown for an Irish girl in a snowstorm.

Oh well, I thought, I'm still trying to do something caring and loving for my husband. "Señor Valdez," I coo, wafting the aroma of coffee all over the house, showing off my new skin. "Come a little bit closer, you're my kind of man, so big and so strong, I'm all alone, and the night is so long." Dear God, please let the reader laugh and know that I am not one of those ladies who greets her husband at the door wearing nothing but Tupperware lids.

So, those were my goals for this time in my life, my mid-forties. At other times, they would be different, perhaps more career oriented, more spiritual, more community based, or financial. Your own goals will or may be different. You may find that the side effects of treatment affect you differently, so your goals may be more about treatment or work. Whatever you choose, the sheer joy of achieving your goals will get that courage muscle working. I don't know why it works, and I wish I could write the kind of book where I could make up a convincing case to prove to you that it does. I only know that every single goal you achieve for a day makes you stronger, and you are going to need to be strong.

YOU ARE WHAT YOU THINK ABOUT:
WHAT'S ALL THIS AGAIN ABOUT A POSITIVE ATTITUDE?

Everyone is going to tell you to have a positive attitude. You'll hear it so often you'll want to scream. But there are mental exercises that will help you a great deal, and you can actually have a positive attitude even if you don't have one now. Unlike that relentless witch who keeps lecturing you about it but is the most negative person you ever met in your whole life.

The Mayo Clinic published an article saying that optimists live longer than pessimists, which of course came as no surprise to either group. The science writer Stephen Jay Gould said that he asked Sir Peter Medawar, a Nobel Prize Winner in immunology, what the best prescription for success against cancer might be. "A sanguine personality," he replied. I look up the word, hoping that it means "sarcastic." Sanguine: cheerful, confident, hopeful, optimistic. I read this and my heart sank. I am many things, I think, but sanguine? Yikes.

I learned how to start having a positive attitude, and here's the trick: you start off by just *pretending*. Start with one half hour. (More than that becomes the strain of being someone you aren't, so start small.) Whenever you see someone, walk briskly with your arms swinging. Smile broadly. Tell them you feel great and mean it. Ask how they are and mean it. Repeat on the next day, and the next. Believe it or not, this works. Eventually, it will become a habit to think positively. Give yourself three weeks to try this and see if it works for you.

Why is it hard to do this? To be brutally honest, I was afraid that everyone would believe me and expect me to be performing at top speed. After all, it is easier to limp around, pale as can be, and let the world pity you. On some days, that's exactly what I did. (It's easy – just go out without make-up. "Oh my God!" people will say. "Has it spread?") But eventually I learned that it didn't matter what other people believed unless they were close to me, and those people knew the details behind the positive attitude. They never deserted me just because I said I felt great. My sister-in-law would say "Are you sticking to that story?" Yes. I am.

The only negative experience I had in telling people "I feel great" was with one person. You know the kind who hates positive people? His favorite quote is "an unexamined life is not worth living?" To which I say, didn't Socrates say that before he drank that hemlock? Don't you think he started thinking then that maybe any old kind of life was worth living? Anyway, this person suggested that I wasn't really doing great, I was just "in denial." I laughed. "I would love to be in denial," I said. "But every time I look in da mirror I remember I got da cancer and da chemotherapy." Normally, anytime I respond to someone in a mean way, God will punish me almost immediately. This time God said, "Let it go, I can't stand him. He reminds me of Socrates."

So the starting point is to use your demeanor to *look* positive, which does help you to *feel* positive. But we both know that a positive attitude doesn't just mean smiling broadly and often. It's a general expectation that things are going to turn out okay, which is a whole lot harder than grinning, because it is based on hope. Hope is, at the same time, both the most essential and the hardest of all human emotions to maintain on a lasting basis.

The ultimate goal is to develop a positive attitude that will feel natural and right. That's the kind of positive thinking that works, and if you feel it inside then how you show it is up to you.

There are a few more exercises that get your positive muscles working.

So far we started by doing a little arm-swinging walking and some smiling. Next, try to fill your mind with active thoughts that are not about cancer. At first, this is just like when someone says to you "Don't think about elephants." I used to carry a small notebook with me so that if I found myself in a situation that could foster lots of negative thoughts I could use my notebook to play word games. A handheld computer works really well, because you can look very important while you play games. During treatment, you may not want long drawn-out mental challenges, but keeping your mind buzzing is very helpful. Try reading a news magazine in a language you don't speak.

Many people feel that the opposite of a buzzing mind is helpful, too, in the form of meditation. My father swears by it and it helped him greatly in dealing with prostate cancer. I can't seem to get the hang of meditation, but I know it works if you like it.

I found that different distractions worked at different times. Sometimes it was being with other people, sometimes it was serious reading, sometimes it was MAD magazine. Some days, I would work hard at something that was challenging, and that would feel great. Some days I would plow through three newspapers, reading every word. Other days I would skip right to the comics. Some days I would pick up free weights and lift until it sank me. Other days it would be Game Boy and a nap. Anything to help you think about something besides cancer for part of every day.

Of course, it helps to think about those seven basic things from elsewhere in the book, when I didn't know what process would strengthen our inner courage muscle. Love of life? Love of children? Love of husbands, wives, partners, family and friends? Prayer? Friendship? Fear of death? Laughter? The more you think about those seven things, the stronger the courage muscle seems to grow, and that's a very good way to think about something besides cancer. Go bowling with an old friend this weekend. Laugh out loud a lot. Go to a movie with your husband. Spend a moment praying deeply. Read something challenging or something fun. Take pictures of your wife and kids, then go to the drugstore, drop off the film, and buy a photo album at the same time. When you pick up the film, sit in the car and put the pictures in the album before you go home. (Nothing makes me feel better – well, morally superior actually — than having pictures in a photo album.) Throw away the negatives if you will never use them and they will make you feel disorganized.

Come up with your own ideas, because mine will sound stupid to you. I know that whenever I read a list like this it always sounds stupid coming from someone else. Cheer myself up by decoupaging my garage door? Please shoot me on my way to the craft store. Plan a romantic dinner and eat naked in the dining room? Too much peanut butter and jelly on those chairs, thanks, they'll never pry us off.

Cancer actually *helps you to think positively.* We had long standing plans to go to Madrid, for the wedding of our dear friends Elena and Carlos, when I was diagnosed. We've known them forever and we'd been planning this trip forever. We went anyway, the next day in fact. I can honestly say it was the best trip ever. Missed flights? Lost luggage? Nothing mattered to me. It was enough to be with my family doing something new. Everything was a source of new enjoyment. And now you know where I got that pitcher of sangria.

Some people call this "living each day as if it were your last." I don't. I even think that is just about the worst philosophy I ever heard, even worse than "love means never having to say you're sorry." The world can't afford to have everyone doing no work at all and sleeping with Paul Newman, which is what I would be doing if it were my last day.

Instead, it's living each day on purpose: very intentionally and mindfully, and if you have the energy, passionately. Doing what matters most. It's as if your alarm went off a little early this morning, and instead of hitting the snooze button you decided to get up and get going. Well, unless you're Joanne Woodward.

Note to self: would those wonderful Make a Wish groups handle adult requests? And just how charitable is Paul Newman?

There is just a little actual scientific proof that a sanguine personality is effective against cancer, but if you could get a group of oncologists together, they would probably agree that people with positive attitudes often fare well.

I hate to write this message, in a way, because it makes it sound as if it is your fault if you're not doing well. The fact is, there are fighters with a strong spirit who are taken by cancer, and there are whiners who survive. I don't want this positive thinking message to become another piece of pressure put on cancer patients to be as perfect and saintly as possible. But doctors do notice that a strong will to live is a good sign in a patient; try it out for yourself and see if it's helpful.

LOOK AROUND

I found it very helpful to become more observant of everything around me. I would really study how other people live their lives and handle challenges. Most of the time I was observing ordinary circumstances, and my favorite place to observe was in the Oncology Department. I would watch the staff and marvel. If I knew that some percentage of the people I met everyday weren't going to make it, I would have to be detached. I could not stand the pain of working in such a place unless I protected my heart against getting too close to people. I expected chemotherapy to be a very cold place.

Instead, the staff was smiling, greeting you like a friend, warm as anything, treatment after treatment. I felt very comfortable there and very welcome. I never figured out how they did it, but it was amazing to watch. When you observe something amazing, doesn't it make you want to be a little amazing, too? When you watch the Olympics, don't you run a little faster the next day? So I would look, and look and look at everyone around me for examples of sheer achievement, and that would help me to strive. People who have worse problems than cancer bringing dinner to *us*. A man I saw over the years walking briskly with his wife and dog; then with just the dog; then alone, but still walking. People in wheelchairs going to work everyday. A couple I see who walk their dog every morning; the combined age of this trio is about 500 years. As slow as the humans are, the dog is just plain glacial. That dog would drive me nuts. It takes them all day, but they do it. Every day, people everywhere get up and pick up a burden, but still do something more today than they would have done had they taken the easy road. You're going to be one of them.

There are so many inspiring people in life. The more you look, the more you find them, the more you learn, the more you achieve, the stronger you get, the better you feel. Take a break for a moment to realize that you are getting stronger, whether you planned to or not.

LOOK WITHIN.

Now we're back to one of the first things you did: think about your own strengths and how they can be used to handle this crisis. Jot down these ideas. Every once in a while read them over and add to them.

TRY A FEW THINGS.

You've listed your strengths and you've set some goals. As time goes by, you'll add some specific goals to your overall ones. Now, meet a few goals and exceed a few expectations this week. Some weeks, for me, meant finishing a major project, but other times it was as simple as watching the news so that I wouldn't withdraw from the world, even though I wanted to.

You're not just having goals so that you come out of this with a few important jobs done. It doesn't really matter if your goal is to paint the house, make yourself a millionaire, get fit, go to church or just clean up the candy under the couch cushion from last Halloween. *The idea of goals is that each one you achieve makes you stronger and makes your courage muscle stronger.*

Does it sound cruel to you to expect yourself to have goals at this time? Yes. But enough good people will pamper you and feel sorry for you. We all do need that, but I love what my wonderful friend Laura did for me.

I had just had my first round of chemotherapy. I spent the day with Laura, which we do sometimes. We tell our husbands that we will be gone for an hour or so, and they love us enough to say "Okay, see you in an hour." As

soon as we leave, they gather the children and begin showing them our pictures so that the kids will remember us when we eventually come back, which
is in a very, very long time.

Laura suggested that we go bowling. This was in tribute to her mother,
who, like mine, died too young of melanoma. On the night when Marian
found out that it was her time to check out, her kids couldn't find her,
because she had gone bowling. It was, after all, her bowling night, and she
saw no reason to miss it. So off we went in her honor.

Laura hammered me. I would remember the score except that it was too
humiliating. I complained to her that I was a cancer patient and she was
being pretty mean.

"You've had exactly one chemo treatment," she said. "*Talk to me when
your hair is falling out.*"

I love that. Laura — who came to treatments, made dinner, listened to
all of my complaints — never changed how she talked to me. It reminded me
that your character doesn't have to weaken just because your body does.

And also, since it's my book: I let her win.

Set a few goals and watch yourself grow stronger. Before you go too far
with this, remember that you are setting reasonable goals.

LATHER, RINSE, REPEAT

I admit it – the most helpful words I have ever heard come from a shampoo
bottle. Lather, rinse, repeat has become my motto when trying something
new. I have tried many new things and quickly learned that some of those
things were really bad ideas, and the only thing you can do is let it go and try
again with something else. I remember thinking that maybe this would be a
good time to – well, fill in the blank. You name it, I thought of it. At first,
when I would stop doing one of these new projects, I would feel terribly
guilty. I'm a quitter, I would think. I can't finish anything. Try a new career?
Take a course? Learn to cook? Learn a skill? Start a business? Learn an instru-

ment? Finally know all the words to any song at all? I've started them all and quit many. Even as I write this book, I know that it may well be another of these ideas.

If it is, I will try to remember what I've learned: New ideas are not contracts or vows. They are experiments. The only absolute vows in life are to finish school, be faithful to your marriage, raise your kids and care for the least among us. Nothing else is eternal, so when you try an experiment and quickly realize that it's wrong, you are better off letting it go than trying to finish it at all costs to your energy and sanity. Let it go and start again tomorrow — Rinse and repeat. So, if your goal this month was that you were going to go to work every day no matter what, and then you got the flu, well, let it go and start again tomorrow. Oh, and drink plenty of fluids.

Your house, after all, is full of unfinished projects. So what? Some people advise you to throw them away, others to finish them all. I say leave them where they are until the day when your kids are cleaning out the house and putting you in a nursing home. Let them deal with it. That's why I had kids. You?

One new thing I did successfully was to manage my treatment days. I went for long treatments on Wednesdays, when I had a full day of babysitting arranged and would not worry if things were behind schedule. But managing means much more than that: it's learning what you really need and fine-tuning that along the way.

For me, sitting in a chair all day during chemo became harder and harder, so I needed to avoid anything passive. Watching TV was out, though I thought it would be great. Wrong. In fact, everything I thought would work didn't. I packed a bag of some favorite things, like a favorite book, crisp apple strudel and cream-colored ponies, but I used none of it. I'm guessing that I did not want to associate my favorite things with chemotherapy, and I didn't realize that I would until I actually got there.

It took me awhile, but I finally came up with my plan, which was *to make good friends sit there and entertain me.*

Today, for example, I invited my local brothers and sisters, four of them, to spend the day. My nurse was enthusiastic about this "chemo party" and made sure that we had room to do it. We had a great time – we realized that it was a rare opportunity to spend time together without our kids or grand-kids, just two brothers and three sisters behind a curtain. It was fabulous and the day flew by. But chemo parties are not for everyone, and some people pre-fer to go through chemo alone or even asleep.

For me, it worked to think about each treatment and decide who I thought would be best to be with. It made my treatment much more bearable. Our original plan was that my husband would be there for every chemo treat-ment. Well, he's a wonderful guy, but he's just plain too worried about cancer and chemotherapy to spend the day playing word games and laughing. We agreed that he would focus his attention where it really counted: appoint-ments, planning, decisions and knowledge. He's great at that. He's not great at word games.

You may find that you want to switch a few assignments, too, after you get some experience.

Back to the point. This is a good time to try new things and let them go when they don't work, especially when it comes to chemo. This isn't a marathon in which any change in the plotted course would be cheating or giv-ing up; I even had a session in which I changed my mind about it right in the middle. I had wanted to try doing one session alone. I thought it was going to be short, because I hadn't paid attention, but it was all day. By noon I realized that this, for me, was a dumb idea. Lather, rinse, repeat. I called my husband. "Drop everything, honey, please. And bring chocolate chip cookies."

REVIEW

Once a week or two, take stock. If you can, do it yourself and then repeat it with your spouse or best friend or therapist. How are you doing? What changes would you like to make? Are there goals you want to abandon? New ones you want to adopt? I enjoyed doing this on Fridays, which seemed to help me forget about it for the weekend.

I mention "therapist" here. Many people find support groups or therapy to be very helpful, because sometimes you need to talk for way more than even your best friend can stand. Sometimes, you also need to learn from other people. I was lucky to know a therapist who had had breast cancer herself and similar treatments. I liked her approach and saw her periodically throughout treatment. It was a great help. She was an inspiration to me as a breast cancer patient. She was one of the people I interviewed who set the standard for me to follow.

Many people swear by groups. Finding the right help is not always easy, so if you need help, and many, many people do, support groups can be a godsend right now. Your hospital or wellness center may already have a very good one going, saving you a whole lot of time, money and research. Plus, you don't have a lot of extra time to go around interviewing. No other profession has a higher number of really awful people in it than therapy, not even hairdressing. If you don't believe me, just ask a therapist, preferably one who is not currently institutionalized.

Whether you go with an individual therapist or a group, it's probably best to stick to people who have oncology experience. You could go broke explaining it all otherwise. *Tell me again what reconstruction is, Mrs. Spencer? Thanks much. Oops, our time is up.*

And, wherever you go, quit going if it is not helping you. Look at a group, see if there are a few people in it who seem great and who may have something to teach you. Otherwise, I'd rather save my energy for myself or my family and friends. One warning: don't take advice about groups from people who are from big families, like me. I am the seventh of eight children. Groups of any kind make me start shaking even if they are doing something I like.

I've written this section specifically about cancer, but it actually works for any long-term challenge. Moving to a new place. Grieving. Living with teenagers, then living without them in an empty house. Any change that requires some long-term shifts in how you live your life will be greatly improved by building the courage muscle within you.

SUMMARY SO FAR You've established some overall goals for most days. You've started reviewing and fine-tuning them weekly or bi-weekly.

A Circle Theory for Coping with Friends and Strangers When You Have Cancer

THERE IS SOMETHING UNIVERSAL about big news in your life. The news can be good or bad, life threatening or joyous. It doesn't matter. Whatever it is, you can be sure that someone you know is going to say something really awful.

New parents tell stories about this all the time. The co-worker who tells horrifying labor stories is just waiting for the baby to be born, because then she can say "Enjoy this now because wait until you see how awful it gets when they are (pick one or all) toddlers, teething, teenagers."

When you are diagnosed with cancer, word will spread quickly in your world at work and at home, and the questions, comments, advice and stories will come rolling in. In the first few weeks after my diagnosis I was stunned, and I asked my chemo nurse if other patients have trouble with this. "Let me know when you think of what to say to people," she said, "because many patients talk about this."

You know how our generation feels about our mother's generation — that they didn't tell anybody about any thing, didn't talk about their cancers, miscarriages, life crises. When I told an older woman I had breast cancer, she said, "Do yourself a favor. Don't tell anybody."

I was stunned and asked her why. This is a tiny, soft grandma with that white hair, those pink cheeks, that soft twinset and pearls, the album of grandchildren carried in her purse. "Because everybody is a f-ing pain in the ass," she said. "Everyone will say, poor you, poor you, and if you ever believe that, you're finished."

There were times when I wished I made it a secret, when I thought our mothers were right. Sometimes it would be nice to go to work or the grocery store and not have to talk about cancer with yet another person who heard. But at the end of the day, I think it's better to be surrounded by people who know than not, as long as you can stand the occasional awful moment.

After enduring a few months of those moments, I tried to understand a little of it. First, I noticed that most of the thoughtless people I ran into fell into five basic categories.

THE END IS NEAR

This person has known at least five people with your exact diagnosis who look just like you and who died at your exact age.

HEAR NO EVIL, SEE NO EVIL, SPEAK NO EVIL

This person says that "there are so many medical advances these days that I'm sure you don't have anything to worry about." End of conversation. Don't bring it up again. Bye.

WHAT DID YOU DO WRONG THAT I DON'T DO?

This person, strangest of all, needs to investigate. One eyebrow goes up as they glare at you. "When was your last physical/mammogram/colonoscopy?" they ask suspiciously. And then: "Do you smoke?" I have learned the only answer to this person. It's to ask them, "By the way, what's a mammogram?"

I KNOW WHAT YOU NEED

This person has a lot of advice to give you, from alternative treatments to what doctor you must be seeing or you are throwing your life away. "Attitude is everything," they will say. "You have to be positive." This is true, but coming from someone who flips out over a parking ticket it's a little tough to take.

YOU ARE NOT AS SICK AS I AM

This person, I don't know why, is usually an aunt. She cannot stand for anyone else to be sick. You tell her that you have cancer. "I'm sure it will be benign," she says. For some reason your cancer spoils her enjoyment of her own troubles. Your first reaction to this person is to run when you see her, but try a different approach: wallow in her troubles. Sympathize. Listen for three minutes. The result: you will always feel better, knowing how well you are doing, plus your illness, unlike hers, does not cause you to talk to everyone you meet about your gas.

After defining these categories – and there are probably more – I had a terrible realization: *I have said every one of these stupid things to someone at some point in my life.* I was stunned, but it was true. How could I have said these things? And why?

I tried to think back — when and to whom I was so thoughtless? I could remember saying things, but couldn't remember the people. So then I thought about people I'm close to who have had cancer and realized ... I had never said those stupid things to people I'm really close to. Hmmmm. I would say: you're such a great person and I hate to hear this is happening to you. How are things going? What can I best do to help out? I'll bring dinner – would tonight or tomorrow night be better? I'm going to pick up your kids and take them out for a few hours. Do you need any rides? Need errands done?

Thinking about this led me to understand why I was not bad with people who are close and terrible with people who are not. It starts with understanding that we are all surrounded by circles of people.

THE CIRCLES

Your life is organized into circles around you, like the rings in a tree. Picture yourself at the center. Go ahead, live a little, be the center of your own universe.

In the first two rings are your family and the people who care most deeply about you. You may not be aware of exactly who is in these inner circles until you have a major event in your life, and you may find that people move in and out of these circles. When you tell these inner circle people about your diagnosis, they are stunned, frightened, saddened and they usually show it. *They care a lot about you, so they put their own needs aside for the moment.* Later on they will think all kinds of things, but right now they are just thinking about you.

In the third circle are the friendly acquaintances. They are co-workers you have lunch with, but never see on weekends. These are people you call friends, until you are planning your daughter's small wedding and realize that they won't be on your list. Or your kids are friends, but you don't get together as couples. Some of these people will be great. If you had another life, they would be in your inner circle. Others in this circle will teach you why you would not ever have them in your inner circle. They will keep moving out and out until they are in a distant circle on another planet.

The circles of people move out farther and farther from you until the last one, which includes all of the people you haven't met.

WHY WE SAY THOUGHTLESS THINGS

When someone in the first circle tells you they have cancer, you are only thinking of them. You care so much that it overrides everything you might be feeling. You never say the wrong thing.

When someone in the eighth circle tells you the same news, *you just plain don't care enough to push your own feelings aside.* Did your mother die of cancer? That will come flooding back, and that's all you'll talk about. Did your best friend refuse to have a physical, only to find a cancer too advanced for treatment two years later? Are you afraid of every lump you feel? Have you been worried lately about those headaches? Whatever is on your mind, that's what will come out of your mouth. Once I realized this, I began to understand why people say so many bizarre things, and to forgive it and them.

That explains the mechanism that allows otherwise nice people to say these things. But then there are always a few not so nice ones, too. I finally understood what happens to them – they are just plain terrified of cancer. They need to figure out how to distance themselves from this news that you have it.

The best lesson about cancer, for me, is first learning who is in the inner circles. Then, it's realizing that when your energy is limited, you devote it to the inner circle people. If you have some energy left over, spend it on someone less fortunate than you. You learn that you don't have the energy to stand at the front door listening to another parent whining about the PTO fees yet again, so you learn to say, "It's so good to have a chance to talk, but I just have to go now." Sometimes those circles of people feel like a stack of hula hoops, all spinning at once, and you have to let a few of them fall to the ground.

Cancer has taken everything and everyone in your life and put it into a big coin sorter. It chugs away, sorting all of the quarters, dimes, nickels and pennies into chutes, and then hands them back to you. You can now see the value of each, and decide whether you will spend your time on your quarters or your pennies. Hint: it's the quarters.

The hard part is that some people will disappoint you. Many cancer patients have stories about close friends they don't see anymore. It's easy to say you're better off without them, but it's harder to deal with the reality. You'll forget them in time, or reconcile, but you'll know which circle they belong in. Often, these are people you've done many favors for in the past. I don't know why.

Another great thing about having cancer is that so many people are really nice to you. Nobody would be mean to a cancer patient, right? It's terrific. And the people who can't bring themselves to be nice to you? They just avoid you. When I realized that, I thought about shaving my head forever.

I heard one piece of advice: to spread a rumor that you are going to leave your insurance policy to all of your friends, because by the time they find out it's not true they will have been really nice to you for your whole life and you'll be dead anyway. I would have done this except that then it wouldn't keep working on my kids. (Just kidding, kids, your inheritance is intact and is not going to be spent on plastic surgery, a year in Italy and gigolos like you heard me jokingly planning with Auntie Laura.)

On the positive side of dealing with people while you have cancer, one benefit of cancer is what it can do for your self-esteem. People laugh at your jokes. All of your ideas are just great – no, fabulous. For all I know, this book is terrible, but nobody will tell me because I have cancer. It's just like being, well, a boss. I know it's not healthy, but I'm going to enjoy every last minute of it. Another reason to keep shaving my head when my hair grows back.

Sometime about halfway through treatment I discovered something that is probably obvious to everyone else: cancer is really tough on your siblings. I'm the youngest girl in a large family. My life growing up consisted of my kid brother and me watching six kids and my parents go through the teenage years before us, so I've spent a lot of time hiding from these people. I have always assumed that they are all nuts, because there were so many years of someone else's puberty in my childhood.

Eventually, from my point of view, Mom put each one into a white dress. She and Dad gathered family and friends and made the sister leave home in a big car with a stranger driving it. The sister left and didn't come back for a long time, so we little ones always assumed that Mom and Dad had finally given up and sent her to an asylum. Which was fine, because in large families nothing matters more than suddenly getting more closet space.

So the first time that one of them choked back a sob when I lost my hair was a shock. I hadn't understood how profound it was for a kid sister to have cancer. There was a lot of joking – bald jokes, dividing the inheritance by seven instead of eight, people asking "what's eating you?," but it was still a very emotional time.

The emotions, like many things in large families, were divided. Eldest: "Mom and Dad were much stricter and poorer in my day. We weren't *allowed* to get cancer."

Middle: "I don't resent you having cancer or anything, it's just that everyone ignored my son's graduation because you were sick. You'll get sick a million times but a person only graduates from kindergarten once you know."

Youngest: "Can I have your old records?"

Perhaps I should worry that my brothers and sisters will read this and be offended, but they'll never see it. The older ones are too busy to read. The middle ones only read self-help books that apply to their spouses. The young ones can't read at all. So this would be a good place to confess that I was the one who ... . Never mind. It's an Irish family. You remember that Irish Spring soap that is manly, yes? It's called Irish because it is made out of nothing but Guinness and old grudges. You learn young not to confess.

How to help your siblings? You don't have to for now, because they are

> TAKE A DEEP BREATH
>
> How would I answer Holly's question now — what do you say when people burden you with so many unhelpful comments?
>
> 1. Take a deep breath and take a moment to remember what circle this person is in.
>
> 2. Is what you actually say. Here's what I came up with: "Oh, enough about me. Tell me how you are. No, really, tell me about you. How is your (job, kids, spouse, whatever)?" This works because it makes you feel like a nice person while at the same time stopping the flow of the talk that can sap your strength a bit.
>
> 3. Lather, rinse, repeat.

more worried about you than about themselves. But remember that they are feeling this very deeply. Keep them in your innermost circles, keep them up-to-date and keep them close. (If you don't have e-mail yet, this would be a good time to get it. It's a great way to keep everybody informed.)

THE BEST THING ABOUT CANCER

Once you figure this whole thing about the circles of your life out for yourself, your treatment year becomes one of incredible discovery about human kindness, friendship and love. You receive kindnesses that are beyond your imagination. Friends will express their affection for you in ways they've never said or done before. It is the most incredible lifeline, to feel deeply loved at a time when you may be scared or sick or both.

You will discover a well of kindness in you, too, that I think is put there by all of the love you receive, with some help from God. It will help you to maintain the hardest human emotion of all, which is hope, which you most need now.

I don't know why love and kindness generates hope in such supply, but it does. And if you start cancer a sophisticated intellectual who hasn't said anything sentimental since junior high, you're going to end it as a greeting card writer. It's the unbeatable part of cancer so you should probably just give in now.

So How Do You Help People in Treatment? Some Golden Rules

HAVE YOU EVER OFFERED TO HELP SOMEONE and wondered why they never take you up on it? Or, someone offers to help you. Is your first response to say thank you but you're fine? Read on.

Ask people what they need most. Dinners? Rides? Babysitting? Errands? A chance to talk? Prayers? Company? Information? Take the kids to the library? Go to the post office?

Listen carefully to the answers and try to respond as closely as possible. Please try not to take it personally if we ask you to do one thing and not another. There are people in this world whom I love dearly but don't ask to drive anywhere, what with them only having a scooter. I sure hope they bring dinner and stay for a visit, though.

If you like to send flowers, and they love flowers, great. Otherwise, try taking the car and cleaning it; try a gift certificate for cleaning the house; for a take-out service; for cleaning the windows. Or send something for the kids, like a new game.

Best way to avoid doing anything to help anybody: When you say "Let me know if I can help, really, call me" you will never, ever be asked to do anything.

MAKE IT EASY FOR THEM TO ACCEPT HELP.

Examples: I've made dinner for you. Would you rather have it tonight or tomorrow? I'd like to have your kids come over for a few hours on Saturday. What time would be good? I'd like to take you to a radiation treatment. Is Monday or Tuesday better? That tip is drawn from what successful salespeople do: give the customer a choice between two positive alternatives.

IF YOU LIKE TO GIVE GOOD ADVICE, BUT YOU HAVE NEVER BEEN IN THE OTHER PERSON'S SHOES, FOLLOW THE GOOD FRIEND'S GOLDEN RULE:

Step 1.   Be quiet.

Step 2.   Listen.

Step 3.   Be quiet again.

Step 4.   Lather, rinse, repeat

... AND ADVICE FOR YOU

ACCEPT HELP, BECAUSE YOU NEED IT.

Quit the "I'm fine" stuff. It's annoying and it reminds everyone of their most martyr-like relative. Let people help. If nothing else, maybe it can give your spouse or kids a break.

ACCEPT HELP, BECAUSE OTHER PEOPLE NEED TO FEEL THAT THEY ARE DOING SOMETHING. THEY CAN'T CURE YOU, BUT IT FEELS GOOD TO DROP OFF DINNER.

Are you the person who is always organizing things? If you are, you already know that it is much easier for you to give than to receive. Receiving someone's offer of help and accepting it is, for you, an act of generosity. That will either make sense to you or not. If it does, do everyone a favor and accept their help.

WHEN THEY HAVE TROUBLES, HELP THEM.

The single most important question you
can ask your doctor:
"What is the procedure for asking a question later,
which is when I will think of it?"

Doctors are from Pluto, Patients are from Goofy: Doctor-Patient Communicating

IT'S YOUR DOCTOR'S TURN TO FANTASIZE. In his or her fantasy, all patients talk like those EMTs on Emergency shows. "I am a Female, 46, cardiac arrest, something left ventricle, something 180 over something." I could fill in those words but that would take something that serious oncology writers like to call "research," which is too hard for me, because it means "staying up late enough to watch ER." Anyway, in the doctor's fantasy, we give them all the essential information they need in one minute, they treat us brilliantly, we all get home in time for the daughter's soccer game.

But here's the reality of the patient conversation: "Well, Doc, I hate to bother you, but the other night I had this pain. Kind of a sharp and dull pain at the same time. It was Tuesday, no let's see it was Wednesday, because it was my bowling night, or maybe it was Monday. Anyhoo, you probably don't want to hear my whole life story, so I'll quit beating around the bush and get down to it. It was Wednesday, which I know because the pain started just after my cousin – well, he's not really my cousin, but he's the son of a really good friend of my parents, and we always called her Aunt, so we just always called him cousin you know what I mean? And that's the side of the family that has diabetes when they get old and stomach troubles when they're young. Of course, they're not really related so I guess that doesn't matter much to you, but you never know. Anyway – the pain started just after my cousin dropped his bowling ball on my foot. Being a doctor and all you can probably see how my foot now points in that funny way toward the window."

If you look carefully, you'll notice that your doctor has now ground his or her teeth down to nothing. He or she has no patience left, and the next few questions will seem just a little cold. So now you think he or she is a little big for his or her britches and he or she could learn a thing or two about his or her goddam little bedside manner.

Did we all miss the day of school where they taught doctors and patients how to talk to each other? I have this new business idea – teaching doctors how to interrupt patients without hurting their feelings, and teaching patients how to ask questions. I think we could save billions of dollars in lost time. And I am as guilty as the next person – rambling on and then being mad when the doctor cuts me off.

Before we go another step, I'll tell you that I'm not trying in this chapter to reform anyone – doctors or patients. I'm trying to stand in each person's shoes to see if that could help make things work a bit better, for all of us who are not already perfect!

I knew I would have trouble communicating with doctors the first time years ago that one told me he was going to "take my vitals." Being a woman, I didn't think I technically *had* "vitals," but being skilled in self-defense, I made sure to take *his* "vitals" first, before I learned that we had just had a slight misunderstanding about what "vitals" are. Sorry, Doc, ha-ha-ha, I'm sure you'll laugh about this someday. The nurses, who knew he was one of those arrogant little interns, were already laughing right that very minute, but that's another story.

Why, Doctor, do we patients do this? Because, you see, *I don't know what you need to know.* I am not rambling because I am lonely or stupid – I'm rambling because I am not a doctor and I am *nervous*. I'm telling you everything unfiltered. I have seen enough soap operas so I know you will cure me based on some obscure thing I said about my bowling night or that I once went to an island off Beri-Beri.

So I need you to *organize this conversation, as warmly as you know how, from the beginning*. Know my name before you walk in the room. Say hello to me and look me in the eye when you do. (Note to residents and interns: be careful here. You have not had much contact with animate people lately and you may look a little creepy when you look them in the eye. If the patient recoils, back up a little. Remember to blink.) Maybe even shake my hand. Note to R and I: this is contraindicated if it's broken.

Summarize why you think I'm here. "You're here because your foot hurts, Ms. Doyle?" If I begin to ramble, step in gently – "let me make sure I get the right picture here – is it your left foot? Right here?" This is a good time to let the patient know who is boss by pressing as hard as possible on the spot that hurts, like you always do.

When I ramble, keep me on track in the same way with a set of "Polite Interrupters." These include: "Let me clarify a few things. Does it hurt here?" "Let me make a note of that and then I have a few questions." "There are a few more things that I need to know before we can decide the next steps." Avoid looking at your watch and saying the same things your spouse hates when you say: "Can you get to the point?"

At some point in medical school they taught you to say "That's helpful to know" when we ramble. We are all on to you now, so quit saying that. It means "What you are telling me is so irrelevant that I'm not even writing it down. I am writing a note to myself to pick me up a six pack and some corn pads on the way home. And by the way you need a therapist."

Next, make sure to connect with me. This is easier than it sounds. You don't have to be my best friend, or even remember me. Just make one observation to every patient that says you have noticed that they are there. There are some doctors who make me want to scream "I'm over here!" I want to play my version of that "what color are my eyes" game that women do when they are really, really mad. "Close your eyes, Doctor. Now tell me something, am I a man or a woman?" You have hundreds of ways to connect with me. You can even just ask me what it's like outside.

I know we expect a lot of you. We want you to treat us as if you care about us personally, but if you really care about every single patient, how can you survive this job? It's one aspect of great medical professionals I'll never figure out.

Enough of the nice talk. My favorite surgeon story is about the brain surgeon at another hospital who was taking care of my dad's subdural hematoma while I was in treatment and still pretty bald. I wanted to know my dad's prognosis, so I asked this doctor. I said "Is this a bump in the road or the end of the road?" He said: "Oh, it's a bump in the road. This isn't something bad, like *cancer*."

My whole family froze in horror. "Ix-nay on the ancer-cay!" I heard someone say. They were all looking at me and shaking their heads at the doctor in disbelief. I have seven brothers and sisters, and being the youngest girl I feel a strong sense of protection from these siblings, so I think he was lucky to escape with his life.

But what a great time we had. The guy started a blush that began in his toes and finished somewhere ten feet above his head. This is a very handsome, 6 foot 4 brain surgeon and he melted into the floor. He apologized about 85 times. My family moved in for the kill. "Sensitivity isn't *brain surgery*, you know." My family, not unlike the hyena, is funniest when there is a victim.

I'm not mentioning his name because this story makes him sound awful, but in fact he was great to my dad and I liked him very much. When a really good doctor has one slip of the tongue, I think you forgive and forget. Well, or put it in a book.

Not being a doctor, not even playing one on TV, I don't really know what they would want from us. My guess is that they'd like us to call about questions in a timely way. Have you ever done the Friday night call? This one must drive doctors nuts. You start feeling sick on Wednesday. You think it will get better. Thursday you're worse, but you still think you might get better. Friday morning you feel a little better, but then Friday afternoon you don't feel so great. Friday night you realize that you're really sick and if you don't call right away you'll never make it through the weekend without an antibiotic to treat your virus. So, from the doctor's point of view, you wait all week and then call when everyone is now home with their families.

They'd like us to stick to the recommended maintenance schedule for pap tests, mammograms, blood pressure, turn your head and cough, etc. etc. They'd like us to take medicine when we're supposed to. They'd like us to call when things go wrong.

Most of all they probably want us to lose weight, quit smoking, exercise regularly and eat a healthy diet. Which we'll all do, starting … tomorrow, which is when they will too.

If you have always had trouble communicating with your doctors, *now is the time to change*. Your days of ignoring everything are unfortunately over. The easiest way to change? BRING SOMEONE WITH YOU. Ask your buddy to help you remember questions and answers. Choose this person wisely. I took my sister Terri once and this was her total recall from an entire day of chemotherapy treatment: "Jeez, your doctor is handsome."

Have a list of questions with you. Your most important question is: *Ask what the procedure is for asking more questions when you think of them later*. Later is when most of us seem to think of our questions, and you want to know what to do. Is there a call-in time? Does the nurse act as a go-between? Do you just call?

Back to fantasies. In our patient's fantasy, Dr. Kildare is walking the beach, a lone figure staring out to sea. "If only I could cure her," he thinks, having thought of nothing but me all day. "I won't rest until I find the answer." His wife has left him – all you care about is that Spencer woman! Her illness has *ruined* our marriage!

He is in agony – "I know I've missed something ... help me cure her, God ... wait a minute! I'VE GOT IT!" he says, racing his sports car back to his parking space right at the front door of the hospital, where I am lying serenely in a neatly-made bed, my gleaming blond hair tied perfectly in a white satin ribbon. "It can't have been caused by your cousin's mother's stomach! The bowling alleys in Beri-Beri are *closed* on Wednesdays!"

He kisses me. I notice for the first time that my doctor looks like ... Paul Newman. But I am married to the Count LaScourge, I say, and he will kill you. Dr. Kildare's hands, burning with a love too intense for the limits of the human heart, gently free the white satin ribbon. Oops, that's a different book. Never mind.

HOW TO HANDLE A WOMAN

What a romantic song that was when I heard it at 13 and lots of other times. "The way to handle a woman, is to love her, love her, love her." Then gorgeous Richard Harris got weird and did that raining cake thing, plus he didn't age so well, though he was wonderful in Harry Potter. Bear with me, I have a point here.

Breast cancer must be tough for both male and female doctors to communicate about. It is so emotionally charged for some patients, not so for others. When I first collected a bunch of materials about it, I was stunned by how relentlessly and stereotypically feminine they were, and those were the ones written by women. The chapter about your tumor's pathology report? Decorated with a flower. Your resource book for state agencies? Enhanced with poetry written in calligraphy. I was waiting for perfume samples to fall out but I guess the raffia bow kept them in.

Life was starting to feel like one long douche commercial. Cue the orchestra, fuzzy up the camera lens, blow some tropical breeze through the sheer silk curtains? Must be time for some feminine hygiene. So some of the professionals, thinking that this must be the way women like to talk, sounded like that to me in the beginning.

I have mixed feelings here. I want medicine to be sensitive for people who need it to be. I just can't stand it when "sensitive" means "stupid." Do you know what I mean? The kind of doctors whose voices go up an octave when they talk to a woman? Especially, and I hate to say this, female doctors? But they don't know it? And they end their sentences as a question?

Do you remember a few years ago when the TV network that had the Olympics decided to "target the female audience?" If you heard one more damn moving story were you going to scream? Did you ever feel more embarrassed to be a woman, or even to know one, in your whole life? Should I stop that annoying question thing now?

Oh my God, people thought, I hope my son doesn't marry himself a woman, 'cuz from what I see they must have mighty awful taste, plus, all they seem to do is figure skate. Anyway, I love an inspiring story as much as the next person, but we have our limits, or soap operas would be on all day on every channel. Sometimes you just want to watch the race. Thank God most horses can't talk. "Well, Mr. Costas, Kentucky is a tough place when you've been gelded … ."

I admit that sometimes I felt the same way about breast cancer communicating. There is a tremendous focus on the emotions involved, especially about breast surgery and reconstruction. I don't like myself for how I feel about this, it's just that to me a lot of people in the breast cancer world treat it as an emotional problem that has medical overtones, when to me it is a medical problem with emotional overtones. I think this is a swing of the pendulum, so it will be fine at some point.

Since this book is about choosing your own way through cancer, I respect the choices everyone makes. But deep down inside, in the dark and mean part of me, I am just a tad judgmental about this. Please don't tell anyone I said so, but there are a few breast cancer madonnas out there. These are people who write endless poetry about their breasts, so I am thankful they didn't get rectal cancer. Oddly, the more emotions a person talks about, the earlier their cancer stage, but I don't know why. I just noticed that it is the more advanced patient who is telling everybody to shut the hell up about her feelings, while the rest of us lesser stages are quilting our emotions into a memory book. And if you want to read some really intense emotions, read some essays by someone who has had solely a negative biopsy. "Touched by Cancer," the essay will be called.

If you don't believe me, check out a few articles that are out there, in which the biopsy process is up there with famine and pestilence. Chapter Two: Victory! Chapter Three: Survival! There was an article in a major weekly newsmagazine this week, written by a woman who had a benign lump. She called this experience "Confronting Breast Cancer." It's her right to write like that, I guess, but what moron of an editor printed it? (Clearly not the kind of brilliant editors who work in the book world.)

How can the reader tell if he or she is in this group, whether a doctor or a patient? Here's a simple test: If right now you are feeling that I am "using valuable energy on negative and non-productive feelings," never mind that I spend all of my waking hours trying to be positive no matter what I get dealt, then – it fits! Buy that shoe!

Phew. That's out of my system. It probably sounds harsh, and I always say you should never put anger in writing, and if you do, you should then throw it away.

So you shoulda seen what I really wrote.

CAN'T I DO IT MY WAY?

If you or anyone you know has ever given birth, you may remember that there was a set of things you were supposed to do. Where I lived at the time, you were supposed to have read about 50 books, joined a support group for new moms, signed up for an infant massage class, dedicated yourself to a drug-free labor and delivery, etc. If you didn't, they were going to tell you at the hospital that you had to go home and do so before they would let you give birth or something.

Ten minutes into it I realized that breast cancer is just the same. Damn.

Here's my problem: I didn't want to spend any extra minutes of my life on cancer. I wanted to put into it just what it needed, no more, no less. If I needed support groups, I would have gone – I think they can be very helpful. I didn't go to wellness programs, seminars or meditation classes, or mind-body connection workshops. People kept bugging me to do these things to relieve stress, but the biggest stress in my life was the people who were bugging me to do these things. I've mentioned elsewhere in this book that a therapist who had breast cancer was a big inspiration and for me that was enough.

I had simple goals. I wanted to continue to live my life as richly as possible during treatment. I wanted to be happy. I found that I could achieve these things on my own, so I could spend any extra time or energy on other things besides cancer.

One of the best people I know has cancer himself. He has benefited from wellness center programs, and so he e-mailed me: "these people are great, if you want to go I'll go with you."

How perfect is that? He never bugged me about it, just gently offered. Through treatment, I would get e-mails from Bill, every one of them inspirational, every one reminding me that I am strong. I loved that. I hope you have someone in your life like him.

Other people, well, they mean well. No matter how cheerful I am, they still have a program I need to make me cheer up. No matter how serene I am, they have an activity I need to do to relieve stress. Cancer patients have to do these things, I was told so many times.

I was just simply and joyfully aware of being Stage 3. Okay, that's not as good as Stage 1, but it beats Stage 4, because, as they say in *Wit*, there is no Stage 5.

When I was 18, I worked in an unusual office overseas. One of the first visitors I saw had leprosy, which was the single most astonishing sight I have ever seen, then or since. At the time I was finishing a long recuperation from a weird case of pneumonia and was too young not to feel sorry for myself. But I remember meeting this man and thinking, now, *that's* a disease. To have your face rearranged forever, to live that way forever. Our beloved friend Marie was diagnosed with Creutzfeldt-Jakob disease. There is a zero survival rate, and the diagnosis is a death sentence. *That's* a disease.

If all goes well, I'll simply put in a year of challenges and then be fine. To be honest, don't people with diabetes have it worse over a lifetime? I'm saying that there's cancer and then there's cancer. I just have cancer, and I'm thankful for that, thankful for the fact that you can survive it pretty well. I'm thankful that I don't have *cancer*. If I ever have *that*, then I'll go to every program there is. If Bill is free.

THE DOCTOR I HATE MOST IN THE WHOLE WORLD

If we all share every detail of our medical lives with each other, we all have met the same doctor or nurse: the one who never seems to believe you. You're in pain? It can't be that bad. Your back is crippling you? That's just stress. You have tremors? You must be nervous. This doctor never wants to prescribe anything or any reason, especially if there is a chance that it might make you comfortable.

I don't know what makes certain doctors this way. I've had a bunch of ideas, but the only common theme I can find is that they are mostly just mean people. If they are young, they are also people who often seem scared to me; they want to talk you out of being sick so that they won't have to take any steps that might backfire or, worst of all, make them look stupid or get them yelled at. This is the nurse who won't wake up the resident for you or the resident who won't page the attending physician.

Here's some evidence that this doctor is also not the brightest crayon in the box: We all know that if you ask these doctors for only Tylenol, they will be willing to give you Percocet. Ask for the Percocet and you will get Tylenol. We have all figured this out, but they haven't. They also think we throw Percocet out when we are finished with the pain, when in fact every woman who has ever had a baby still has three Percocet in a bottle and will never, ever, throw them out, and will even be buried with the bottle, "just in case, you never know."

I actually think that this doctor does not last long in oncology and that you are unlikely to have this happen. But if you do, please remember that you truly can't afford to tolerate him or her when you are being treated for cancer. Here's a recommended script: "Doctor, for some reason you don't seem to believe me when I have pain. I'm wondering why, but mainly I'd like to hear a good plan for managing side effects." You cannot allow yourself to be in any more discomfort than necessary, because your body needs to be as strong as possible and as unburdened as possible to fight cancer.

Some of us have trouble having these conversations with our doctors, or anyone else on the planet for that matter. So many people seem to be able to have tough conversations with anybody, but I'm not one of them. If a salesperson has been helpful to me, I can't even return something that turns out to be broken. I make my husband do it, which he doesn't want to do either, so he says "My wife made me return this."

If you have trouble having this conversation with your doctor, and you can't find one that's any better, then the problem, unfortunately, is still yours and still has to be fixed. You may have that unreasonable fear of having an adult conversation with doctors, which I have. Doctors may as well stand on a street corner and ask me if I have any spare change, that's how much I want to talk to them.

You have to be in good shape. So if you can't just suck it up and talk, remember to bring a buddy with you who will help.

ALTERNATIVE MEDICINE AND COMMUNICATING

Are you being treated at a hospital by oncologists? Then at some point in your treatment, someone is going to ask you why you're not choosing an alternative route. "Traditional medicine is hidebound in Western thinking," they will say. "It is tied to the money machine of American culture. Nobody can make money off of natural remedies, so they only give you things they can patent. If you were in Sweden, you could be cured because they don't care about money and they would give you this new treatment from eggplants. And you wouldn't be throwing up like that. Eeew. Well, glad I could help. Bye."

Here's what I say now: "I looked at many methods of treating cancer and the best track record seems to be with this treatment." As you know from this book, all I really did was drink a pitcher of sangria and smoke a cigar. However, I did read a few magazine articles about Suzanne Sommers trying an alternative treatment, so that counts. And I am almost positive that the cigar was made from organic tobacco and the sangria was sulfite-free.

I believe that there are effective treatments outside of scientific medicine, which haven't been tested enough to understand their efficacy. Acupuncture seems to be a proven pain reliever; meditation seems to relieve stress; I know that aromatherapy can help me to feel awake; our friend gave me a Reiki treatment and it felt great.

COWARDS DIE MANY TIMES BEFORE THEIR DEATHS; THE VALIANT NEVER TASTE OF DEATH BUT ONCE.

Speech on the Ides of March by Shakespeare's Julius Caesar, who, valiant or not, probably should have planned to stay home that day anyway.

I like the rest of the speech too:

OF ALL THE WONDERS THAT I YET HAVE HEARD. IT SEEMS TO ME MOST STRANGE THAT MEN SHOULD FEAR; SEEING THAT DEATH, A NECESSARY END, WILL COME WHEN IT WILL COME.

I feel sure that cancer treatment can be aided by alternative ideas. I like my doctor to be familiar with these and not to laugh about them unless he can cure what's wrong with me. Can't get rid of my back pain? Then do me a favor and shut up if my chiropractor does. Can't cure my insomnia? Then don't sniff at my meditation classes.

In return, I won't expect you to prescribe things you can't be sure of.

Keep an open mind about them, but explain to me that you can only treat me with things that have been proven to work and to be safe, and that Wart that belonged to St. Joseph isn't on that list yet.

I saw a documentary about parents with terminally ill children. The parents are telling the doctor that they heard about Treatment XYZ and would like to look into it and ask what he thinks. You know what the doctor said? "My time is too limited." Their 12-year-old is dying but the doctor's time is too limited?

Could this otherwise good doctor really mean to say that? To be fair to doctors, here's what we've done to them. We've put them through the most grueling education we could come up with. We trained them to rely on science and what can be proven so that they are not experimenting with human beings as guinea pigs. First, do no harm, their oath says, which is a dramatic, powerful thing. Not second or third, but *first* do no harm.

But now we are saying to them that we *want* them to believe in things that haven't been proven yet. Give them to us now. But wait — don't treat us like human guinea pigs or we will sue you. We won't be suing the people who promote unsafe "natural" remedies, because they put that little FDA sentence on every bottle that covers their asses. And at the same time doctors know full well that charlatans out there are ready to prey on any desperate cancer patient who comes near.

Example? I came across a web site for an alternative cancer treatment. They start with a profile of people who survive cancer. "Skepticism about conventional medicine" is high on the list. Plus all sorts of squishy qualities that, if I actually have, then maybe an early death is not such a bad thing. As far as I could tell, the only thing they were going to do was listen to my needs, so it's a good thing they care so deeply about me. Too deeply to treat me with any medicine, and apparently too deeply to expose me to the vagaries of health insurance companies, because they won't accept any and by the way they want $7,000 up front. And here's a list of nearby motels you can stay at while we "treat" you.

While I believe in many treatments, my choice was for a doctor to review it all. Many helpful friends told me to take "natural" estrogen from the health food store, on hearing that you get kicked into early menopause by chemotherapy. Since my tumor is estrogen receptive, that would be a terrible idea, because my tumor can't tell if the estrogen is from a health food store or not. On my own, I would have done it, since I am one of those people who tends to believe that anything from the health food store is good for me, and since the employees in that section do not know enough about cancer to understand the harmful possibilities of estrogen for certain cancers.

What I want, and what I think most people want, is a knowledgeable doctor who cares whether I am doing well or not, and will try to keep me as comfortable as possible. All doctors know that nearly every complaint we have will get better on its own with no treatment at all. I know that too, but if you can help me to avoid some pain or sickness, please do, and please use everything you know about.

Here are some things I wish the doctor had said to the parents of that sick child, and what I would like him to say to me:

WE ALL WANT TO FIND A CURE, SO OF COURSE I LOOK AT EVERY IDEA OUT THERE. I CAN'T OFFER YOU ANYTHING THAT HAS NOT BEEN PROVEN TO BE SAFE AND EFFECTIVE – ESPECIALLY SAFE. But I'll tell you what I know about them so that you can make an informed decision. Sometimes it's difficult because there are many dishonest people out there selling empty promises.

I'M FAMILIAR WITH THE TREATMENT YOU'RE TALKING ABOUT. In this case, I don't think it is going to help you because it is an old idea in a new label, and it's going to take you away from treatment at an important time.

Here's what I wish about alternative medicine: I wish the manufacturers would get together and fund research into their own claims. They are not exactly non-profit companies, which you'll see very quickly as you shop around.

And, if I were in medical marketing, I would try really hard to get rid of the word "chemotherapy," which is a pretty unappealing product name that must have been invented in those old World Fair days when we loved chemicals. They must have started out calling it something like AlmostPoisonTherapy so that the chemo name seemed like a real marketing hit.

More advice about dealing with your doctor. For some reason, when you have a serious illness the really good doctors are all really attractive. I thought that was amazing. Then I realized how much we see them through our vulnerable selves, because I caught myself saying that "all doctors are really good looking," and then realized, so how come none of the ones I dated were? (Note to old dates: wondering if this means you? Of course.) Go ahead, enjoy yourself and think they're all good-looking, you'll eventually figure it out for yourself and get over it. (Note to my kids: I'm just kidding, because I didn't date anyone before I married Daddy.)

Have to go. Dr. Kildare, played as always in this fantasy by Paul Newman, has come to my room to see me. I am afraid of no man, he is saying, least of all the Count LaScourge. He takes me into his powerful arms, so strong that I can feel his heartbeat, his passion coursing through every muscle, until the rhythm of my own passion is matching his with every beat of our pounding hearts. But I digress.

A FOND NOTE TO THE FRONT DESK

You have no idea how important you are. You are the first people we meet. You set the tone for our whole experience. So when you look us in the eye and say Good Morning with a smile, you become part of the cure. Every bit of contact you have with a patient counts. Maybe at every other doctor's office we go to, they don't look up, they just stick out a hand for our card and say "Yes?" as if we are interrupting them. If you connect with us instead, if just for a second, you are helping the whole effort.

And you shall love the Lord your God
with all your heart and with all your soul
and with all your might.

—Deuteronomy 6:4-9

In Which I Break Up With God

I ALWAYS THOUGHT OF MYSELF AS SOMEONE with faith, until a series of events in my life, including cancer, began to overtake my abilities to cope. I began having some major disagreements with God and the way He runs His universe.

I began thinking about all of the ways in which it could be done more efficiently and more effectively. Frankly, any one of us could do better. What if the universe were run by the same people who run Disney World, except for the lines?

You don't even have to go that high, because the average transient carnival runs more smoothly and with a lot more fairness than God runs His universe. And I was once on a Soviet-era Russian "cruise" ship with WWII borscht rations that was much more fun.

Why I still refer to God as "He:" any thought I had of God being female ended in childbirth.

So one day I say to God, "I'm not saying I don't love you, I'm just saying that I think we need a break from each other. It's not you, God, it's me. Can we just be friends? I'm not saying I don't love you, I'm just saying that I'm not speaking to you just now."

People began saying helpful things. My favorite is "God looks down from heaven for the broadest shoulders to place burdens on." This comment is always said by very small people, you know, who actually made this up hoping as usual that big people will pick up the slack. Anyway, I would say, next time you're talking to God, please tell him that these shoulders do not signify strength. They signify *being big.* Or, as my best friend says, "God looked down for the broadest shoulders and you were bending over at the time."

People also say "What does not kill me makes me stronger." If you're reading this book carefully you'll recall that this was first said by Nietzsche. However true this inspiration may be, it is still useful to remember that Nietzsche was stone cold dead at 56.

I began quarreling with God all the time. At this point, we were like junior high girls with a new argument every day. Admittedly, it was a one way argument, since God does not answer any of my e-mails directly. Every night, I could almost hear my mother asking me as she once did every night, "Have you said your prayers?" The only prayer I could think of was "Dear God. Thanks a pantload. See you tomorrow." My mother, in heaven and hearing this prayer, did not think it was funny.

How about you? Do you believe in an afterlife? If so, how do you picture it?

I run through all the jokes: I don't want to go to heaven because I won't know anybody. I would miss my friends too much.

But here's what I really see.

I picture myself standing at heaven's gate, on what I think is a cloud. It is really a trap door that leads straight to hell.

I stand there and God says, "Well."

Then He says, "My, My, My." And, in case anyone missed it, "My, My, My, My, My."

He pauses for an eon or two, being a very patient guy, and says "Well, would you Look. Who's. Here."

God looks to His left and right for approval of this bon mot from his colleagues, who all laugh. They are, down to the last one, yes-angels. I realize that I may be in a teeny bit of trouble.

"Guess we enjoyed those seventies, didn't we?" Here I'm thinking that I'm okay, because He said "we."

"Did we meet somewhere?" I ask.

I dodge a lightning bolt. "You are not funny," he says. "Click," goes the trap door, down I fly into hell, and on the way down I can still hear God, who is saying, "Now, you take that Lucille Ball. *She's* funny." The people who sit at the right and left hand of God are saying "Yes, Sir!" just like Ed McMahon and are laughing like crazy. The trapdoor has a way of making them all agree, I guess.

Many people, on being diagnosed with cancer, ask "Why Me?" I don't blame you if you wonder that. Other people will say that oh, they never asked that question, because they refused to indulge in self-pity. I can't stand those people, can you?

I never asked that question "Why Me?" either, but that's because I already knew the answer: God thinks I deserve it. He puts these burdens on me because he just can't stand me. That's the real reason God puts burdens on any of us. He just doesn't like us. Poor Job.

One great thing about Job is that both Christians and Jews refer to him in times of trouble. Religious people in both groups tell you to read the Book of Job when things are tough, because there you will read about why bad things happen to good people. As far as I can figure out, the meaning of Job is that if you keep a dung heap in your yard, and you go and lie down on it, you are 100 percent certain to get sores, so don't go blaming them on God. But at least it gives us something ecumenical to agree on.

After two years of distance from my faith, I felt a yearning one night to read the Psalms. Not the newly translated Psalms, but good old-fashioned King James nothing-shall-I-want. I didn't know why, but I spent an evening reading from cover to cover. I spent a little time dwelling on the 23rd Psalm, of course, which is so beautifully written, plus I remember Cary Grant praying it in *The Bishop's Wife* and he just looked so great, God forgive me.

At this point I had been feeling that my use of humor in bad situations might not be so great given how often it seemed to irritate people. But I stumbled over the psalm about "Make a joyful noise unto the Lord," and I felt better. Hmmm. I still felt as if I'd missed something as I read, but I didn't know what.

The next day, the phone rings, and it's my niece Christine. I have not spoken with her in too long and in the meantime she has seen sadness far worse than mine. She is a person of extraordinary faith, and I share my feelings with her. She offers me the thought that God led me to the Psalms. I start to joke ... if God is so worried about my reading habits could you suggest to Him that it might be a better use of His time to do something about *cancer*? She laughs and very gently leads me back to the topic at hand.

Listen to David, she says, who is *furious* with God. In nearly every Psalm he is screaming about his enemies, his being forsaken by God, his stranding in the desert, and on and on, and then he ends the Psalm with something like "And by the way God I trust you and I love you." God is trying to tell you something, Aunt Nicky, she says. "He understands that you are angry with Him and He knows that you love Him and try to do His work in this world. That's what matters to Him."

I'm not so sure that anything I do is God's work. By this point I am crying my head off and then Christine finishes me off. "And about that laughter," she says. "God gave you your personality. Don't ever, ever be ashamed of it."

I am crying again as I write this, from the sheer emotion of feeling loved by God, through all of the people who have prayed for me and cared for me, and humored me and comforted me. I begin to see all of the ways in which everyone's prayers have been answered for me, especially the prayer for strength. The prayer for Paul Newman to drop into my lap with some time on his hands goes unanswered as yet, but I am praying for patience.

For now, I actually feel a physical sense of a burden being lifted from me through everyone's prayer. Everyone has put my name in prayer groups and is praying like crazy, and I can actually feel that. For a skeptic this is an amazing feeling, to have a palpable sense of being physically carried. I remember very precisely when the feeling started, and it was a distinct and sharp transition. It was the difference between treading water on your own or sitting in a life raft. I didn't understand the power of prayer until this happened. This feeling of lightness was followed closely by a strong sense of unworthiness. Don't waste all this prayer on me! Pray for other things! And that was followed by a feeling that I'm going to have to live up to all this prayer, and where on earth will I find the energy to do that?

For the first time in my life, I finally get that stupid expression "Don't cross that bridge until you get to it." So for now, I'll just believe that I'll have the energy I need when I need it.

In the meantime, I'm still mad about a few things, God. But by the way I trust you and I love you.

> What man actually needs is not a tensionless state but rather the striving and struggling for some goal worthy of him. What he needs is not the discharge of tension at any cost, but the call of a potential meaning waiting to be fulfilled by him.
>
> —Viktor Frankl, Holocaust survivor
> Man's Search for Meaning

Your Body's Daily Life During The Treatment Year

THERE ARE A LOT OF BOOKS, ARTICLES AND WEB SITES about handling treatment, and your oncologist and oncology nurse are the best sources of information. But like everybody who writes about cancer, I can't resist putting in my own advice.

WHAT DO YOU NEED TO KNOW ABOUT TREATMENTS?

Most books about any subject have been written when the author has already finished going through something. Time begins to erase the more humiliating moments. Do you remember your husband's cut that needed stitches? Not quite the way he remembers it, which is "I got a little cut this weekend. It was no big deal but my wife insisted I go to the emergency room. Needed so much work we were there for seven hours." He was John Wayne.

You remember mostly his screaming, lots of screaming. He begged you to call 911. The injury was so small that you were the lowest priority at the emergency room, behind that guy who's gone there every day for the past eleven years because he was attacked by Martians. You spent six and a half hours in a chair waiting, 15 minutes parking the car and 15 minutes while John Wayne got five stitches.

To be fair, how do you remember childbirth? I remember sitting in a neatly made bed, wearing a satin bed jacket. My sleek blond hair is tied up in a white ribbon. It is a beautiful and tender moment.

That's not how my husband remembers it. But this is my book, so we'll leave it at that. Let's just say that his memory makes him shudder and then he has to go take a nap. Also, I wasn't blond. Yet.

So now that I'm finished with treatment, I can tell you how well I handled it. I felt great, I'll say. I remember sitting in a neatly made bed, wearing a satin bed jacket. My blond hair is tied up in a matching ribbon … . You get the idea. So when someone says, "I felt a little under the weather during radiation, so I sipped on some mint and elderberry tea and felt completely fine," drink that with a really big grain of salt. On the other hand, if someone tells you that they went to bed for the whole time, sprinkle salt on that, too.

The truth is, every day is different, every treatment can be different, every person is different. It took me two treatments before I felt that I knew what would happen. At that point there would be only two treatments left before a different stage would start. I had days that I felt terrific, lots and lots of days like that. Seriously, and so will you. But I had other days when I thought that the gates of hell were yawning open just below my dangling feet. There were very, very few like that. And after a few days like that, I learned that *you are supposed to call when you feel that way. And that's pretty much the most important thing you need to know.*

I was home for a few days feeling unable to get up. I would drag myself out of bed, take the kids to school, and crash on the couch, unable to make it back up the stairs to bed. I tried to go to a store I go to all the time, and I couldn't remember how to get there. This gave me the hint that maybe I shouldn't exactly be driving.

I finally called the doctor. He told me to come in and I said I'd try to get in tomorrow. He said no, he'd see me right now. My doctor is a great man, but he looks like Charlton Heston. So I pictured him sitting with a rifle resting on his lap when he told me to come in now, and so I did. My neighbor drove me over, they asked me a few questions, they hooked up an IV, and 30 minutes later … I felt fabulous. Turns out that I was dehydrated and my blood pressure had dropped. I hadn't noticed that I had no saliva. In future treatments, I would know to watch this carefully, and would come in for hydration before it got bad, because I could drink and drink and drink at home, and not make a dent. I just wish I had called on day one instead of day four. Damn dirty apes.

Saliva was a good indicator. For the first time since I was 12 I had to make sure I could spit. To be sure I was hydrated I therefore visited many tall buildings, but it's still not as fun when you have your front teeth, and I am truly, truly sorry to that bride having her picture taken in front of the Empire State Building.

Dehydration for me was worsened by, well, not to put too fine a point on it, diarrhea. Having traveled a bit, I considered myself kind of an expert on the subject. My sister and I combine information about diarrhea from every continent except Antarctica. Colette favors a case she got while traveling in the neighborhood of the Amazon, after drinking a local beverage made of *spit* in a place picturesquely named "Anaconda Island," obviously by an extremely bitter young man who resented spending his summers there with Grandma. Colette had to be flown out and later produced a worm one-foot long, which is still pretty much the family record, to my knowledge. I prefer a case from the medina in Marrakesh, where I ate a pie containing a pigeon, a bird I would not even walk near but had to try because it is a local specialty. Flying rats, I call them when at home, but "a delicacy" while traveling. Then there was the octopus in a disreputable nightclub in Tokyo, from which I hurt so much that the hospital thought I had appendicitis. The goat brain I nibbled on as an appetizer. The fish stomach for breakfast. The late-night noodle stall in Hong Kong, where you dip your communal chopsticks in tea to clean them, and for which I want to apologize to that ladies room attendant, to whom I introduced myself as Meryl Streep.

Those were my personal life records. Treatment matched them but did not beat them, but that dehydration was the pits. Throughout treatment, anything that really bothered me was caused by dehydration. I'm telling you about it because it is so preventable, so if you get like this, call.

One day, dehydration made my heart dance a drunken little jig. This was harmless but it sure didn't feel like it, and it was a weekend, which everyone knows is the worst possible time to be sick, except for a Friday afternoon in the summer or in whatever month when those residents are all starting their new assignments. The young cardiologist who saw me does not know that I heard him tell someone that this was his *first* call. I felt that I deserved some sort of prize for not faking a really big heart attack just for him.

Anyway, the staff at the hospital was terrific and I have no horror stories. Everything went professionally, efficiently, and well. I learned yet another great thing about chemotherapy, which is that when you show up at the emergency room with a ticker complaint you don't exactly wait long.

And then I met a nurse whom I should probably not identify, because he might be embarrassed, so I will just give you a hint that he looks like the kind of guy whose name might be Dwayne.

We chatted as he hooked up an IV. It turned out that his wife was at the movies with their young son. I said gee, that's where I'm supposed to be right now. And he said: "Were you taking your *grandchildren* to the movies?"

There was an awkward pause. I had several points to make to this young man, which I always find works better if you get their attention by first wrapping the IV tube around their ears, which takes a minute because they have those little stools on wheels which makes them a little hard to catch.

I gave him two gentle pieces of advice. The first was to go F himself. So was the second.

If you're a grandma you probably wonder why I'm so darn sensitive. I wouldn't have been, maybe, if I hadn't been called "Sir" that morning, plus I'm only in my forties, so Grandma was now too much. And I wouldn't tell this story if this guy not named Dwayne but with a name that is spelled just like it, hadn't been such a great nurse. But he was, so I get to.

Anyway, your doctor and nurse will go over treatment side effects and what to do about them. I had mild side effects but acted as if they were major so that my husband would do all of the chores. This is what is known in treatment as a "coping strategy."

You'll find your own way through which side effects bother you. Paclitaxel chemotherapy gave me some intense muscle pain, but I could cope with it since it only lasts a few days, and the doctor gave me good pain relief. I didn't get the numbness that some people get until after the very last treatment, but then it lasted for a hundred years or so. Cytoxan and Adriamycin gave me the dehydration, some queasiness and a few mouth sores, and all chemo gave me yeast rashes on my alabaster behind, which you treat with the same stuff you used on your babies. Well, technically it wasn't my alabaster "behind," more like my "front."

And of course everything gave me diarrhea and then fatigue. They treat that with over-the-counter medicine and then give you tips for taking care of your tender bottom, including using baby wipes and baby diaper rash cream. You haven't lived until you've shopped up and down the baby aisle while you're having a really good hot flash.

Chemotherapy is hard, but it's not the horror of old. Survivors from those days must look at us today and laugh, if they have stopped throwing up yet. There are many medicines to help with nausea, pain, anemia, mouth sores, and so on. The point is, if you're feeling lousy, *call*. They'll do everything they can to help. That's everything you need to know, because by the time this book is published, there will be even more anti-nausea, anti-pain, anti-fatigue help available. It's not the old days, and you deserve some help and some relief.

SHALL I RING UP THOSE BRAS FOR YOU, SIR?
(DECIDING WHAT TO DO ABOUT THOSE NO HAIR DAYS)

Men look great bald, totally bald. I never saw a bad-looking guy in chemo, because men just look great bald. When a guy has cancer, he can buy a few caps to keep his head warm, but otherwise his appearance, frankly, actually improves. He may look a little green, he may get a little thin, but there's still a Yul Brynner thing going on.

You probably know that it's the chemotherapy, not the cancer, that makes you bald. Not all types cause baldness, but many do. Chemo attacks all cells, not just cancer cells, and it affects all of your fast growing cells, like where hair grows. And not just on your head, if you catch my drift, which I really liked because you feel so minty fresh all the time. Perversely, I lost hair everyplace except my legs.

Anyway, women also look great bald, but you'd never know it. The first thing many women do before they start chemotherapy is start buying hats and wigs. I did that too. I spent a lot of money very quickly, even though it was against how I wanted to approach this.

I had decided that I was not going to hide my head. I thought about painting it, decorating it. People e-mailed me ideas – paint it like a bowling ball. Paint a globe on it. Paint a face on it and pretend you're walking backwards. Paint it like a bottom so you can moon people. I began telling everyone that I was going to be publicly, unabashedly, bald. And then I ran up against the most formidable objection possible: my nine-year old's feelings. I was reminded for the thousandth time that you don't have cancer by yourself.

Do you remember being nine or thereabouts? Do you remember your mother having the most embarrassing raincoat, or hat, or something? Now picture your giant mother bald, picking you up at school. Not a happy, happy thought.

Wait, I'm getting ahead of myself. I had had my first treatment and we were going to be at our family reunion in Arizona for my-mother-in-law's birthday. I had packed a wig and some hats just in case, since we were going to be posing for family pictures, but I had already made a decision. When the hair started to come out, I would shave it off. Some people say that this is psychologically easier than losing it gradually, but I had only one reason – I hate housework and I was not going to spend one minute cleaning up hair around the house.

Midway through our trip, my hair came out in clumps. Jeanne, the mother-in-law everyone dreams of, offered to take me with her to her salon for the shaving. She was amazing. You would think that every day of the week she took someone to have their head shaved, that she often went twice a day or so, that she had been taking people for *years* to have their heads shaved, so comfortable did she seem with the whole idea. And when it was over? "You," she said, "have a really pretty head." She is a national treasure.

Jeanne's stylist sat me in the most public chair. I offered to move back to a private area if she was uncomfortable with this. "I'll move if you're uncomfortable," she said. "Otherwise I'll tell everyone you lost a bet. Now, let's have some fun," she said, and shaved a stripe down the middle of my head.

It is not an easy thing to have your head shaved, but Judi made it hilarious. It was a tad traumatic, but fun. I learned a wonderful lesson, that some people will rise to the occasion when you have cancer, and they will make you feel great.

Back to my life as a mom. I decided that knowing your mom has cancer was enough to deal with, and that I would wear the wig around my daughter's school. Gradually, I switched to a hat. Even more gradually, I switched to nothing when we were around town on errands, but I never went bald to school. That was our deal, and I stuck to it. For her part, Katherine did more chores around the house than any nine-year old in history. She would go, humming, just as my mother always did when she cleaned, and I would listen and smile, and I could feel my mother smiling too.

The kids at school were all still curious about why I wore hats, and I told them that "I was taking a special kind of medicine, not the kind that you take when you're sick, but a different kind, and it makes your hair fall out! It will grow back, but I have to take this medicine for awhile, so it's going to take some time." They got used to it.

Money saving tip: Before you go shopping for a wig or hats, ask your chemo nurse if they have any donated ones. I bet they do. Or, consider buying a cheap wig but having your own stylist do it for you from time to time. Makes all the difference.

The point of this chapter, like this whole book, is to tell you to do whatever you feel like doing about your hair. Like a wig? Great. Like the Orthodox snood look? Great. Prefer Mr. Clean? Great. Want to go African with fabulous turbans? Great. Your hair does not have to be something you spend a lot of courage on unless you want to. I've met women who never left the house without a wig, because in their world everybody is always perfectly coifed. Go ahead and do that, even though your daughter wants you to "be yourself and go bald." Perfectly coifed is yourself, and that's your choice.

If I could send only one message to every cancer patient and your families and friends, it would probably be about that: you have to choose your own way through treatment. Anybody else's way is just going to be a source of stress, because the strain of being someone you aren't is major. So if you are a perfectly coifed, perfectly manicured, perfectly dressed person, then be that person. Your daughter-in-law's insistence that you are hidebound to society's opinion is just that, an opinion. I hope that she will have the grace to keep it to herself, even though you have three wigs that are all exactly the same. And if you are a well-coifed woman's daughter-in-law, who wouldn't wear a wig even if it were made by a rain forest women's collective out of recycled Birkenstocks, then your choice to go baldly forth is your choice, too.

Now, life is short, and you love each other, right? So maybe you could think about doing something nice for each other from time to time. When your daughter-in-law invites you to a teach-in on breast cancer, leave the wig in the car and have a ball. When your mother-in-law invites you for lunch with her friends, put on a wig, and again, have a ball. But compromise in everyday life? No. That's for *you.*

Why the title to this section? Because I am sometimes called Sir when I go about my bald errands, and I'm used to it. Today, it was the guy at the bookstore where I bought Lance Armstrong's book. One night, my husband and I took an evening out, and the bartender said "What would you gentlemen like to drink?" I laughed, leaned over and kissed my husband as passionately as I know how, which is saying something, if I have to say so myself. Even if I'm a man, he's the guy for me.

I never thought I'd be in the position of offering beauty advice, and if you saw me you'd laugh at the very idea. But if you want to look great, pay attention to your coloring and your eyes. I never did figure out liquid eyeliner, but I did find that if you use a pencil and a smudger tool that it looks pretty good when your eyelashes are missing. Eyebrows can be brushed on with practice, or there are stencils you can buy and dab them on. I tried false eyelashes but never wore them. A little blush and a little lipstick will give you some color when you have that lovely grey look from chemotherapy. Put the lipstick on first to keep you from putting too much blush on.

As my hair grew back I decided that it looked kind of good, so I had it neatened up as it grew out. I stopped hiding the fact that my hair was already white when I was in my thirties. Chemotherapy made me a combination of Punk Rocker and Judi Dench, and I thoroughly enjoyed that. I would never, ever have had the guts to cut my hair this short and it was fun to try out a whole different image. I'm thinking of keeping it for good.

AS YOU GO THROUGH EACH STAGE OF TREATMENT, SEEK INFORMATION ON COMFORT MEASURES.

People who had cancer years ago marvel at the many advances in comfort during treatment, so take advantage of everything there is. Mouth sores? Nausea? Diarrhea? Anemia/Fatigue? Pain? Call your doctor or nurse, because the medical care you receive as a cancer patient is amazing. You just plain won't believe it. For your first treatment, they'll give you the measures that work for most people. Then they'll fine-tune it. You'll think of your doctor as a very, very attentive sommelier of an incredible cellar of drugs. You've always suspected that doctors are holding something out on us? That there are secret medicines for every little discomfort? You were right. So call.

People also like looking up information on side effects. On the minor side, I did not have much nausea *caused* by chemotherapy, but I had nausea caused by the *thought* of chemotherapy. Only a fellow cancer patient would believe me. As I got in the car on the morning of chemo, I would feel sicker and sicker, so that by the time we arrived I would be the kind of green that I thought was reserved for pregnancy or a pigeon dinner in Marrakesh. Bob Champion, the jockey who went on to win the Grand National, talked about this continuing for years after treatment whenever he got near the hospital.

Anyway, anti-nausea medicine didn't wipe out this particular kind of loony-tune nausea for me. Then Marge, from Nature's Gift, an online aromatherapy business, sent me some ginger in a bottle. Sip it, sniff it, she said, I've heard it helps. Well, it did. I mentioned it to my obstetrician neighbor who said that pregnant women drink it as tea and that it helps them.

Do yourself a big favor: before you try *anything*, ask your doctor about it. Ask the doctor who knows the most about the appropriate stage of treatment; if the comfort idea is about surgery recovery, ask the surgeon, etc. Which reminds me that telling specialty doctors what other specialty doctors think about something is just good, clean fun, because it turns out that they all think other doctors are *idiots*.

Try it out. "Umm, Dr. Smith Phlebotomist? Dr. Jones Surgeon said that he thinks this problem might be caused by the something of the something." At this point Dr. Smith smiles one of those smiles that means this: "that putz." Then she will explain why Dr. Jones is insanely wrong, but she will start her explanation by saying "With all due respect to my good friend and colleague Dr. Jones … ."

And to the friend who wanted to know how I could be so nuts as to be bothered by nausea that was all in my mind? I'm sorry I threw up on your cat's favorite chair. And that cat is ugly.

A CANCER THING I'D NEVER HEARD OF.

Sometime after surgery, I started receiving a lot of compliments. People would look puzzled, look at me very closely and say, "Do you know you look great?" At first I thought it was my new breasts, admittedly the cutest in the known world. But I'm lying in bed, recovering from pretty significant surgery, in a hospital – and feeling, well, a little bit absolutely terrific. Everyone started commenting on it. Eventually, I said something to my oncologist. "I don't understand why, but I feel better during treatment than I did a year ago."

I assumed it was my imagination, but he had seen this before. A person's body is fighting the cancer for a long time, and the byproduct of that fight is feeling lousy. You don't know that's what it is, because you don't have any actual signs of cancer yet. I remember complaining about fatigue, but I thought that was middle age approaching, which of course it wasn't, not by a long shot, me being so darn young and all. I was getting more and more sedentary, which meant that I gained more weight, and soon developed sleep apnea, which makes you feel the same way you feel when there is a newborn in the house who expects to be fed all night long and you are the only one who will admit to having a working pair of breasts.

When the cancer is removed, the body can stop fighting and go back to its normal jobs. The difference for me was astonishing. So if you've been feeling terrible for awhile, pay attention after surgery and see if this might happen to you. It feels *great*.

IS IT THE SIXTIES AGAIN?

Once or twice during cancer treatment they gave me drugs that were, well, kind of fun. I'm not a drug fan, or even an alcohol fan, so I hated some aspects of these experiences. Mainly I hated that they had to end.

Before you take Paclitaxel, or example, they give you some really big doses of steroids. This made me high as a kite and it lasted for a day or two, I think. My favorite memory is looking at the time and realizing that by 7:00 a.m. I had done my walk, done a step exercise tape, finished the grocery shopping and worn my husband to a frazzle if you know what I mean. The only awful part was that they crash you in the middle while you're actually receiving the Paclitaxel, but that's okay because you'll be heading up again in a few hours. They explained this to me carefully and there are some really good reasons for it, but I was way too high to pay attention, which felt very familiar and is the same reason I can't tell you much about Microeconomics 101 or 102, except for one complicated formula that I memorized to the tune of Black Magic Woman. Note to my kids and to Professor McCarthy: I am just kidding. It was In-A-Gadda-Da-Vida.

On this subject, I found that pain management has changed a great deal since the last time I had surgery, mainly now they actually give you some. They used to think that every single patient would become addicted to painkillers, but that was before they knew that the expression "addicted to painkillers" is used by celebrities because it sounds so much better, and more crime-free, than the truth, which is "addicted to cocaine." The current think- ing is that people *in pain* don't tend to become addicted to painkillers. So are you thinking of toughing it out because you "don't want to become depend- ent?" For most people that's not going to happen. You probably make everyone miserable when you're in pain anyway, so do yourself a favor and get some relief.

Have you experienced those patient-driven pain things yet? They give you a button and when you push it gives you a little painkiller. They encour- age you to stay ahead of pain so you can go ahead and push it every 7 minutes or something like that.

Some people love this. I thought it was stupid. I work at forgetting about pain. So? So I forget to push the button. A couple of hours go by, I now want to get up for a walk down the hall. It has been ages since I remembered to push the button, so now the pain is pretty bad.

The nurses who took care of me were great, but when I explained this problem to the nurse on duty that day, her advice was that I should "watch the clock." Is it me, or is that nuts? I should lie in my bed and watch the clock so that every 7 minutes I can push a button? I generally try to treat everybody with courtesy, but by now it was a strain.

On the next round of doctor's visits, a wonderful young resident listened to my story. Within minutes the stupid button was gone and they gave me pills on a schedule. I know that a lot of people like those buttons. It just didn't work for me. If you have the same experience, remember that you do have options.

WAKE ME UP WHEN IT'S OVER: FATIGUE

I admit to being the world's biggest baby when it comes to fatigue. It doesn't have to be caused by treatment, it can be any old kind of fatigue. If you have the kind of fatigue caused by anemia, be sure to check this out with your doctor for some relief. If you have the other kind and find a cure, please let me know.

Fatigue gets to me. I start feeling depressed, irritable, fearful and hopeless. I find comfort in Vince Lombardi's line about it ("Fatigue makes cowards of us all.") and I've been repeating that to myself whenever I'm tired since I was 21 years old. (I also like "The Green Bay Packers never lost a game. They just ran out of time.")

I think everyone in treatment gets some degree of fatigue. A few things you might want to try:

BE VERY MINDFUL OF YOUR ENERGY LEVEL. Learn to recognize that you are fatigued, so that you can recognize the emotions that go along with it for what they are. They are the evil voice of fatigue talking, not that I hear voices or anything.

SCHEDULE YOUR DAYS AROUND YOUR HIGHEST PRIORITIES, MATCHING THE HIGH PRIORITIES WITH YOUR HIGHEST EXPECTED ENERGY TIMES. Yet another great thing about cancer: you learn how to run your life in a way that works the best anyway.

REST WHEN YOU NEED TO. Sounds obvious, doesn't it, but you really have to do it. No more staying up after everyone goes to bed.

TRY A COOL OR COLD SHOWER INSTEAD OF A HOT ONE. If you can stand it, it helps you to feel more awake. I also found aromatherapy oils to be helpful, which no one believes, but it's true. I use grapefruit oil, spearmint and pine, all over the house, in my office, in my car. It helps me feel awake.

TELL YOUR DOCTOR. Fatigue has a few different causes, some of which can be eased, such as chemo-related anemia. I thought I just had fatigue when I was severely dehydrated, an easily fixable problem.

Most of all, I learned to get things done whenever I had energy. It took some time for me to get into this routine; in the beginning it reminded me of "take your naps when the baby is napping," which makes so much sense but is hell anyway. Work projects, holiday shopping, the kids, the house; I would do anything that had a deadline enough in advance so that if I ended up fatigued it wouldn't matter. Everything else I delegated or forgot about.

Michael makes Thanksgiving dinner, which he loves to do, but I'm supposed to set a beautiful table for it, which I did when I had the energy. I did it in September. I used my remaining energy to yell at everyone not to touch it until Thanksgiving. I would stop yelling now that it's January except that it's already set for St. Patrick's Day.

My standards for holidays did slip a tad. I was hoping that cancer would relieve me of all responsibility for Christmas and Chanukah, but the damn Internet has made everybody think that shopping is now "easy," so that didn't work. Perhaps it wasn't the best idea to use AssortedDeluxeGorgonzolaLiqueurs.com for "Baby's First Christmas" gifts, but isn't it the thought that counts? And was it really that offensive to send my hospital gowns to be used as Halloween costumes for my nieces and nephews next year? Kids love 'em! And what is the difference between that pink bucket of toiletries that is coincidentally given free to hospital patients and a fancy packaged "hostess gift" basket from a store? Are we so shallow? Have we lost the true meaning of the holidays?

Back to fatigue. Did you have the kind of upbringing in which illness was considered a character flaw of some kind? Do you secretly believe it was probably that same character flaw that killed those Mayflower ancestors of yours, not to make any particular ethnic associations with this whole subject or anything? Or do you come from any other place where this attitude exists? Again, and let's be very clear about this, that we're not making any ethnic associations or anything, but did you learn this from your mither? And when they tell you to drink plenty of liquids, do they need to be very, very specific with you?

Then be especially careful about fatigue and side effects in general. When they tell you to call if your temperature hits 100.5, do. Barfing? Call. Sores? Call. Diarrhea? Call. Pain? Call. Have I repeated myself enough for you? Call.

IF I GO TO THAT WEDDING DO I HAVE TO WEAR CLOTHES?

Before surgery you may want to give some thought to what clothes you can wear during recovery. As you slowly start to get out and about, you'll still find that some clothes are easier than others to wear. With breast surgery, lifting your arms is hard; an over-the-head top is impossible, so I needed a few things. All of my nightgowns, both of them, for example, were over-the-head, so I shopped for pajamas. I discovered that very few manufacturers are think-ing of the woman who reaches for the record in both height and breadth. There was exactly one pair available. It was bright orange, relieved by stripes of dark orange. It was about a foot too short and the button placket was crooked.

I looked insane.

Some of the breast cancer books tell you to "tuck" a few pretty things in your suitcase for the hospital. None of my clothes "tuck" very well, given their relative size. So I just had these pajamas that looked like what you have to wear in prison if you are extra bad.

I wore them anyway. Between the baldness and those pajamas, com-bined with my usual loafers with no socks, most visitors didn't stay long. I wore them for one of my first walks outside, and you could hear the shades being drawn and the children being called inside.

RADIATION

I've noticed that many cancer books have lots of information on chemotherapy but not much on radiation. This might be because radiation is one part of cancer treatment that you have to be a whole lot smarter than I am to understand. In this treatment, an invisible beam is aimed at you and destroys cancer cells. In my version, some really smart physicists realized long ago that even other doctors are not smart enough to understand radiation. Grasping the earning potential of such a treatment, they made the whole thing up.

I can see them all now, laughing so hard that they all pee their pants, which is how they invented pocket protectors. They came up with the whole invisible beam thing, knowing that no one will ever figure it out because it's just too complicated. This may sound crazy, but the only other thing I can think of is that they have magic radioactive beans.

Anyway, radiation may be part of your treatment. Just as with chemotherapy, be careful reading general information. If you go online and read a description of general side effects from radiation, you're going to think it will kill you. It turns out that each part of the body will have its own set of side effects. In breast cancer, the most common ones are fatigue and a sunburn on the breast. Be sure you're reading about your own cancer so you won't be really surprised when you develop a prostate sunburn instead of a breast one.

What's radiation like? The first step is a planning session, in which you go to a simulator that looks like the real radiation machine but isn't. You lie down on a table with the body part exposed, so you'll probably be changing into a hospital "gown," a word assigned by somebody with a Cinderella complex and a pathetic fantasy life.

There is a big open L-shaped thing that rotates around the table. They line up some beams of light at precise points on your body, then they put permanent marks there that are really teeny pinpoint tattoos. Some people think it's painless; I thought it hurt, but only for a second. This planning session took about an hour. It has a space age kind of feeling. You can ask the planners if you can choose your own tattoo, ha-ha, but it turns out that every single patient before you has already asked that, even the ones who are not funny.

For breast cancer, you rest your arms above your head in these padded stirrup-like gadgets, so you look like that Goya duo of paintings of the Naked Maja and the Clothed Maja. You'll be looking more like the Naked Maja. Look it up for goodness sake, at least these girls knew a thing or two about keeping their strength up. You can tell they would be ready for any fasting that might be necessary so they made sure to keep a strict schedule of tapas.

Anyway, it's not comfortable but it's not painful or anything. I can only imagine what they use for prostate cancer, but if there are stirrups involved it's probably kind of funny.

You then receive information about what you can and can't do during the radiation weeks, which might be no antiperspirants or powder in the area, which means you will have a hard time telling which is a radiation side effect and which is just a rash from not being able to use powder. They'll give you instructions for your particular treatment. Mine could have been enclosed in a fortune cookie: "You will spend all of your time trying to find a non-antiperspirant deodorant that actually works for you, but you will not succeed."

The table you lie on moves around slowly while they are adjusting you. They use little handheld devices that look like remote controls except they never lose them. It feels very steady. The radiation comes from the big L-shaped thing that they move around you to get it into position. It's not a claustrophobic thing like the various scans. When everything is all set they leave the room, close a really big door, and turn on the beam. You can't see it or feel it, though sometimes people report feeling a tingle. I felt that once, but basically you don't feel or see a thing. I expected it to look and sound like a ray gun so I was very disappointed.

You typically go for radiation every weekday for a certain number of treatments, in my case 28. This takes about 6 weeks when you add in weekends and holidays. You're in the actual treatment room for about 15 minutes or so. They get you into position using the tattoos, then they all leave the room, because in the wonderful irony that is cancer treatment, radiation can give you cancer if you get too much of it. A buzzer goes off meaning that the radiation beam is on. It takes a minute or so for each treatment. In my case there were three treatments in each session. During this time they can see you on cameras and hear you. You don't know they can hear you until you realize you've been singing "Ground Control to Major Tong" and they come in humming it and someone says "It's *Tom*."

They turn off the beam and come back in, by which time the radiation has magically dispersed. They wink knowingly at each other. Sure it has dispersed, they are thinking, because it was never there.

They'll tell you 80 times that this treatment cannot make you radioactive, but I still went into a dark closet to double-check if I glowed in the dark. Our town gets frequent power failures and I thought about the convenience of moving around the house by the light of my breasts, gliding along like the figurehead on a ship. Disappointed again.

I learned on my first day not to get up too quickly from the table, because it turns out that it can move kind of high off the floor. You're better off waiting until they lower it before you hop off. "Hop off" is my cruel way of saying "get up from a position you've held for 15 minutes at your age in which all of your joints stiffened and you almost fell asleep. Good luck. Liftoff."

Every other day I would have "spa day," in which they want to increase the radiation dose to the skin. To do this, they basically try to attract the beam to the skin. It doesn't take much to attract it. They take a wet towel wrapped in plastic wrap, honestly, and put it on you. When they leave the room you feel strangely like a gelatin salad left in the church fridge after a potluck supper.

I learned other interesting things, like why everybody who is going to touch a patient's skin has cold hands. This is because they have a bucket of ice outside the door, which they stick their hands in before they touch you. Nobody knows why, except that this is "tradition." I maybe shouldn't write such a thing because there are people who will take it seriously. With my luck it will be those people who design the devices used in gynecology, who are always looking for new ways to make the experience as unpleasant as possible. Sometimes medicine feels that way, doesn't it? Have you ever had a diabetes test? How long did it take to find a way to make sugar taste that bad? I took one sip. I told them I thought this was the most incompetent and cruelest thing I ever tasted, that I was going over to Mrs. Field's, where they *understand* sugar, and I would be back as soon as I had eaten enough to feel sick. Sadly, this doesn't work.

For me, the fatigue side effect built up very gradually, but it was real. It was not consistent for me, so I had good days and bad days. Usually I felt fine until late afternoon. If I had something to do at night, I would take a nap first. I found that exercise became increasingly difficult and I eventually had to take a break from it. Today, I went to radiation, then to a meeting and did a little work. By three o'clock I was staggering to bed. Now it is two in the morning and I can't sleep. Last week, I had a fully productive and very busy week. But by Friday night I went to bed and didn't get up until Monday morning.

The sunburn wasn't too bad until the end, especially given that my chest is the only part of me that has never been sunburned, except for that one day on that deserted beach, when I was 19, and which I stoutly deny so it doesn't count, and the only witness has mysteriously disappeared. The sunburn did start to get itchy, for which they gave me a cream. While you're in position, you get a little stiff, but you don't have to hold your breath like you do for an x-ray. Every once in awhile they take an actual x-ray while they are giving a treatment.

By the last week, I was looking quite well done. The sunburn was as bad as a sunburn. I thought it was pretty bad. It continues for awhile after radiation ends, even worsens a bit, and then of course it peels. If you have been a sunbather before radiation, the very idea that this stuff is what causes sunburn will probably cure you of it.

In my case, radiation came at the end of treatment. I was getting pretty impatient to be done with it all, at the beginning of the long six weeks of daily doses. Fortunately, I was saved by friends who brought me every day and kept me company in the waiting room, and by the radiation therapists, who were unforgettable. Trivia questions on the ceiling, knowing just how you need everything to be, they were really gifted at this.

As I started each new kind of treatment, I had the usual important questions, mainly, "what can I do to amuse myself here?" I recommend playing freeze tag with your radiation team, not that you should tell them about it. You're kind of uncomfortable on the table, which they know, so they move around doing their stuff at about the speed of light to do this whole thing as quickly and efficiently as possible, which I really like. But they are also very focused on patient care, so if you start to ask a question, they all freeze in their tracks and listen. All of a sudden you're ten years old, it's freeze tag time, and you're it. So, I recommend lying there and every once in awhile just say "Um."

Watch the whole team stop, breathlessly waiting for your question.

"Never mind," you say.

Off they buzz at light speed again. Wait another minute. Then "Um" them again.

This is just one of those favorite hospital games, right up there with "Call Patient Information to see how you're doing."

People say that they develop friendships with other radiation patients because you are there every day with the same crew. I had a different experience, partly because I had company every day and partly because radiation re-united me with my childhood in an incredible way. On my first day, I checked in to see the nurse, who, unbelievably, lived about ten houses away growing up. Donna and I went to the same school from 1st grade through 8th. When I saw Donna there I just wanted to hug her, so I did. I mean, I knew that the radiation oncologist is supposed to be one of those experts and all, but here was a fellow Flagg Street school pal. *That* meant something.

I already said that radiation is one of those fields for really smart people who can understand physics. What I love about cancer treatment nowadays is that these — well, rocket scientists — have learned the human touch. They seem to care so much about your comfort and your feelings that you can't help but wonder if space travel wouldn't be a whole lot more advanced if physicists and engineers had started thinking like this a long time ago. These people would never have allowed those cramped upside down capsules, no. They would have designed the first La-Z-Boy capsule and we would all be going to Mars for spring break by now.

That's how I experienced these people. The department did things I especially loved: free parking at the door, ice water and snacks, the trivia questions above the radiation table and good music of all types in the room. These sound like small details, but when you go everyday they get bigger and bigger.

There is something about radiation that is hard, but I couldn't define it. Is it the going everyday, or the radiation itself, or that solitary moment when everyone leaves the room? I just know that I found that having company made an enormous difference.

I started by going to radiation on my own. My husband came to the first session, then my plan was to stop by for radiation as I was doing other things. After the first week, Michael told me that my friend Jane had organized friends to take me. They would pick me up, wait with me in the waiting room, then take me home. I don't know why Michael and Jane decided this was necessary but they were right. Thank God for Jane, because she did it all.

It completely changed how I felt about going. I didn't even know it was hard to go until I learned how easy it was with friends. It was precious time in busy lives, to spend a little time with people I really like. It was also a way to feel some connection between your real life and your cancer life. It meant more to me than I ever would have imagined, so much so that the thought of it is making tears stream down my face as I write. It was another time of feeling so loved that you just know everything is going to be fine.

I guess I just learned what made the difference.

Anyway, like everything else with cancer treatment, your response to radiation will be individual. Some pretty chickenish people think it's a picnic, some strong people really struggle with it. As always, this is the time to be closely in touch with your team about your own reaction.

For me, I learned why doctors and patients have such different definitions of words, and this helped me a lot. Take the word "fatigue." We all use our words based on our personal experiences. To the patient, we have felt fatigue ranging from a little tired to really tired. A doctor, though, has seen fatigue ranging from a little tired to, well, actually dead. So when a doctor says "mild" fatigue, they're calling it mild compared to being deceased, when it is really hard to get moving.

To me, "mild fatigue" means "not actually tired but kind of bored." It is used to describe that feeling on Holy Thursday or Yom Kippur if the house of worship is a little chilly and you are just a little sleepy. So, if I went to bed on Friday night, and got up on Monday morning, I wouldn't call that "mild." But to a doctor, they ask you a few questions and decide that that seems kind of a normal response. Another good reason to make sure you're both on the same page.

I'm writing this with just three more days of radiation to go. On my first day, the weeks ahead seemed to stretch out infinitely. For me, the warmth of the staff and the pleasure of having company made the weeks fly by. I'll miss the team who cared for me so well here but I can't wait to be done at the same time. It is December and I'm hoping that the sunburn will ease up so I can do some topless caroling. See "Found A Peanut."

Your House's Daily Life During The Treatment Year

THIS MORNING I SAW YET ANOTHER ARTICLE about an amazing cancer superstar. Maybe you are one of those people and you're reading this while you make your own soap or something. Anyway, she runs a business, chairs a few hundred charities, takes care of a few sick friends, and the interview takes place in her "immaculate home."

Oh. My. God.

I have deep respect for people with immaculate homes, I really do. Every two weeks, after the cleaners come, my house is immaculate too. Then school lets out. Here the kids come with their friends.

I will do anything to hang on to this immaculate house, short of actually cleaning it, so I have finely honed housekeeping strategies. I have drawn the shades. Check. I have changed the house number. Check. I have unplugged the phone. Check. I have locked the front ... the one thing I forgot. I race to the door and throw myself against it, but they have sheer numbers on their side and force their way in. "Nice try with the house number, Mom," they say, dropping their exploding backpacks on the floor, next to the 30 pairs of shoes that must wait by the front door, so that they are ready to wear and so that they can hide the pile of overdue library books. My inner witch begins to boil. "I gave you life, you little ingrates, and maybe it's time to take it back," my witch thinks, but I don't let her say this for now.

I've seen quite a bit of advice about managing daily life while you have cancer. This is my favorite: *"ask your older children to assume chores while you are recovering from treatment."* Trot this one out in the chemo area and watch the older parents roar.

Somebody has been watching way, way too many after school specials. When you were a teenager, did you ever once say yes the first forty times your parents asked you to do a chore? So, somehow, while recovering from treatment, I've got to train my teenager to say yes to new chores sometime this year?

So what's the answer? Simple. All parents know that the only way to get kids to do chores easily is to make the *younger* ones do it. Don't waste your time on those hateful teenagers. Use your energy there to best advantage by making them feel guilty. "This was my grandmother's favorite mop during the war. I was going to leave it to you when I ... ."

Focus your energies instead on turning those really little, pliant children into your little helpers. They can do exactly half of every single job you do, except using power tools. They can take out most of the garbage, empty the dishwasher at least as high as the counter, collect clothes for laundry, feed pets. Read up on your Dickens if you don't believe that small children can do chores. They can do all kinds of things if only we force them to.

Now the chores are under control enough for Step 2, which is to "ask" your spouse do the other half. I would love to be the kind of person who "asks" people to do chores. I just don't have time. Here are my timesaving tips.

If you are a man, just tell your spouse you're thinking of taking early retirement so that you'll have more time to do the chores. Your spouse thinks, hmmmm, "twice the husband, half the income" and starts taking out that garbage lickety split. All of a sudden she will know exactly when your car needs to have its check-up.

If you are a woman, threaten to take away the most effective thing you could threaten, which, being a feminist, I am too ashamed to admit that I would do but I think you know what I mean. If you are partners of the same gender, these techniques still apply.

I joke about housework, but it's actually a big deal for me. Once upon a time, I worked full time and I married a man who already knew his way around a kitchen, which I didn't. We divvied up the chores evenly. I looked around and saw that it was good.

Then I decided to spend more time at home with our children, and I learned the painful truth. Unless you have one of the five jobs in the world that are actually difficult, it is way, way, way harder being home. I've lived both lives, and I know why men were keeping that secret from women for so long. The office is a picnic, and the more senior you are, the bigger picnic it is. You know who you are. If someone makes your lunch reservations for you, you would last about an hour being home full time.

That's how long I lasted. I am still mostly doing it, but I long ago knew in my heart that I would never actually be any good at this job. My only talent is creating Things to Avoid Wasting Time, which I am really good at. Hate searching for scissors, tape, etc.? Buy your own private tools and hide them. I have scissors and tape hidden in every room in my house. Hate being the one everyone turns to when they're looking for something? Just refuse to tell anyone you know where that something is. Refuse to answer "Honey, do you know where my keys are?" This tip not only saves you tons of time, it also makes everyone aware of just how scary your domestic power is. Wait until he's old enough to be looking for his glasses and you'll know what power really is.

My next favorite bit of cancer advice is *"Relax your high standards for housekeeping."* I already have the lowest possible standards for housework. When I read about early American life, I skip past the democracy stuff but I am enchanted by one thing: dirt floors. Aaaaah, I think, now *that's* good interior design. There's somebody who's thinking ahead. I'd never have to wash a floor in my whole life, plus everyone knows that you can't keep those kids clean when they're crawling around in the dirt. Laundry? Forget that, everyone knows it's a waste of time. Brush everybody off and let's peaceably assemble or something.

Years ago I told a story to my employer who is therefore just the best, most wonderful person in the world, and by the way I am not writing any of this on company time or on a company computer. Anyway, we returned from vacation to find that the police had been at our home. Our alarm had gone off. Here's what they said: "It's really strange. They didn't take anything but *they ransacked the house.*"

If you are a kindred spirit, you guessed it. The house was exactly how I had left it in the frenzy of packing, but to the trained criminal eye it had been ransacked. I thought this was pretty hilarious and made the mistake of telling it to Alan, thinking he would laugh too.

He was not laughing. He looked me in the eye in that steely way employers and people with immaculate houses do sometimes and told me that "you should never tell that story again."

Please keep in mind that Alan is a wonderful man. But in this moment I realized that there are terrible divides in human society, deeper than race or creed or sexual orientation, and they all involve housework.

What is your point, you may wonder, if you're still paying attention? My point is that you're going to receive a lot of advice from people on handling daily life, but you're going to have to figure it out for yourself, because nobody else's way is right for you. Are you happiest when your linens are ironed and your house smells freshly cleaned? Then do that. Does the car need to be on a strict maintenance schedule or you feel terrible? Do that. Are you not that way? Take the advice of my friend's mother, Priscilla: leave a broom and dustpan out at all times. When you have visitors, say, "oh, I was just sweeping up." I have had a broom out since I heard this story.

Anyway, if you relax your high standards without making someone else do the work, you'll probably regret it. If you can afford a cleaner, now's the time. Otherwise, the time for figuring out how to get everybody to do the job is long overdue. Just know that you won't be able to do all of it all the time. So just teach that little kid to wear oven mitts when he irons.

Speaking of overdue – you know what I'm going to say, don't you? Has your local video store taken out a lien on your house until you return 'Mary Kate and Ashley Clone Themselves at the Dude Ranch'? Have you paid them so much money in overdue fees that they hug you when you come in and valet park your car? They love you at the video store, because you pay them a lot of money and never actually watch any of the movies, so they earn money without any actual wear and tear on the merchandise, plus you save them shelf space.

You learn a lot about your shopping habits when you begin telling people that you have cancer. You learn quickly that the people who care the most about your prognosis are business owners. The video store? The hairdresser? That donut guy? These are the people who *really* care. Your parish priest doesn't recognize you, but the lady at Bloomingdale's knows you down to your underwear. These people are really, *really* worried that you might not make it. When these people say they are praying for you, they really, really mean it. Maybe *they* would do your housework.

Like everything else in your treatment year, ask yourself who you are, because this is no time to use energy being somebody you're not. If you really care about the house, then organize your life and your family to keep it in good shape. If not, well, follow Priscilla's advice. And don't trip over that broom.

In Which I Discover Topless Ironing: Some Novel Ways To Get Used To Your New Body

AT ONE POINT AFTER MY SURGERY, I had to have some bandages changed twice a day that had to be professionally done. (Don't be concerned, that's not typical.) Fortunately, nurses came to the house to do it. Unfortunately, scheduling visits around your normal life isn't always simple. I would take my shower and now my bandages would be soaking wet. I would not want to put a shirt on, so I would be topless for a while as I waited for the nurse to arrive.

One day, instead of sitting around in my room, I did some ironing for one of the kids. Haven't ironed in a generation or so, but I did that day. The next day I did some more, and the next day. I bought a real iron instead of my $15 model and kept on going.

I thought this topless ironing was kind of funny. Oddly dangerous with my new powerful steam iron, but funny. I started doing other topless things,

"I'VE SEEN THEM BURY PEOPLE WHO LOOKED BETTER THAN THAT."
An expression from the Yiddish,
which came to mind in the mirror one morning.

like writing this book. I started doing topless weightlifting. One day, I read in Dear Abby a letter from a neighbor complaining about a woman who walks around her house topless. That's me! I thought, proudly, feeling like a celebrity. Go ahead, Abby! Tell them to MYOB!

I had chosen to have breast reduction surgery on my right breast when I was having my mastectomy on my left breast. This way, my left breast reconstruction would match a newer, smaller right side breast. I love my new breasts. Some people try to make as few changes as possible, given the perceived trauma of new breasts and cancer. That's a solid point of view if you have it, but I didn't feel that way. When the first doctor gently talked with me about many women needing to mourn the loss of a breast, I said, "Stop right there. I have had big breasts forever. Take them off, and make me 16 years old again. Make them so high that I am choking on them." Except for the choking part, they agreed.

I went for my first appointment with my reconstruction surgeon and was waiting for him. Outside his office were his nurse, his office staff, and a high school kid doing some filing for him. After a few minutes, the high school kid came in, shook my hand, and said, "Hello. I'm Your Doctor."

I called him Doogie. I showed him which of my skin rashes were actually older than he is. I asked him if he gave up his career as a Backstreet Boy to become a doctor. "I don't know who that is," he said. My heart was in my shoes. He's not even old enough to know the name of a boy band, or maybe he's a recluse, I whispered to my husband.

I also noticed that all of the surgeons who do mastectomies, taking your breast off, were women. All of the surgeons who make new breasts were men. I knew that I had one of the best breast surgeons in the country doing the mastectomy. How would this young guy measure up?

So the first thing I did after surgery, anxiously, was look at my new breasts. They were … adorable.

Beautiful.

Frankly, they were pert. Even perky.

Firm.

Uplifted.

Porcelain, with a rosy hint of springtime blush.

Ripe with the promise of newfound lust.

(Note to Paul Newman: every word of this is true.)

I wish I could show you how great they are, but I have had to limit such displays to those in the medical profession at my husband's request. I showed them to everyone who came into my room in the hospital and Michael began complaining. "That was not a nurse, that was the janitor," he would say. "That was the billing department. That was your dinner being brought. That was the florist. Oh, My God, that was the rabbi." Anyway, I'm very selective now, so if Paul Newman comes knocking, he's going to have to have a bona fide medical reason to see them. Yep.

If you prefer not to have too much change in your life, by all means opt to have your reconstructed breast look like it used to, as much as is possible. For me, I loved the idea of *newness*.

So, relative youth in a doctor can be a good thing, youth meaning "someone who is not that much younger than me but somehow does not remember the night the Beatles were on Ed Sullivan." This doctor also gave me one of my Top Ten Biggest Laughs of cancer. He was debriding a small section of my back, a charming procedure which I cannot believe anyone can do without barfing once. Hardened war surgeons, just returned from tending the wounded from the Charge of the Light Brigade, still say "Eeeeeew." (Again, this experience is not typical.) I asked him if surgeons were people who could always look at gross things, or if anything ever gave him the willies. "Oh yes, we get the willies," he said, with his knife in my back. "That's why I keep my eyes closed."

My choice for surgery was to have everything done at once, the breast reduction, the mastectomy and the reconstruction. This was because I hated the idea of surgery, it scared me, and I wanted it done at once. See Chapter

2 for more about this issue.

I can't honestly say that I would do it differently now, because you could never have persuaded me back then. My only previous experiences with surgery were awful. One was so bad that I have locked the memory in a little box someplace and never remembered to tell the surgeons about it when they asked for a medical history. It involved the charity ward in a hospital in Hong Kong in the 1970s, no anesthesia and conditions that no one on earth should have to put up with. It left me with a burning rage about the differences in medical care between the rich and the poor, along with my strong distaste for surgery. And a deep and abiding love for the kindness between humans in distress; I will always remember the woman who gave up her bed for me, because my frame could not fit on the little cot they gave me; and the young woman who brought me a book in English. I had been living in Hong Kong for three weeks at the time and could not communicate with anybody in that ward, but these acts of kindness touched me so deeply. When I later experienced the private and rich side of medical care in Hong Kong with a case of pneumonia, it made me a darn communist.

Your new body, even with a terrific surgeon, is going to be different from your old. Some women are miserably unhappy about that. I just think it's a great idea to think about the breasts you want and go for it. I know people who have used the opportunity to go big, or to go small, with great results. If your surgeon isn't interested in making you happy about this, for God's sake just find another one. It is biologically impossible to hurt the feelings of a surgeon, because everyone knows they have all of their feelings except confidence removed after they are certified. If you don't believe me just ask any surgical resident if that's true of the attending physician.

My interest in exchanging my old breasts for new ones helped me to get used to a few things. You're going to have scars. Guaranteed. You're going to have numbness, under the arm, in the breast. If you hate scars or numbness, this is going to be a tough adjustment for you. Don't let my own enthusiasm take away from that; it's going to be an adjustment and you need to give yourself time.

When I mentioned the debridement I had, I skipped over the fact that I had some tissue loss that was kind of gross for awhile. It was, gaily, Kelly green. I've never met anybody else who had this happen so it doesn't seem that useful to go into much detail. I mention it to tell you that yes, I did have days of looking in the mirror and not knowing who that was looking back. One thing that helped me a lot: being thankful that my cancer was in a part of the body that you don't actually need, and I would rather have breast cancer than have it in my liver.

Like chocolate, of course, all of this is related to sex. I'm tempted to offer my own scientific advice for getting used to your new body, which is: buy some Astroglide, have sex as soon as you can after surgery, and enjoy the newness. Iron a little, have a little more sex, have a little more sex, and pretty soon you'll be used to it. Your spouse may be very hesitant about sex at first out of fear of hurting you; you'll have to engage in a long and complicated series of conversations to get him or her into bed. If your partner is a man, and I mean this in the nicest possible way, "Honey, I'm fine" usually works.

But many, many people don't feel like having sex while they have cancer, for so many reasons. If that's how you feel, don't fight that if it would be a major effort. I really hate cancer books or pregnancy books that urge you to "maintain your healthy sex life" as if you have some kind of obligation to do so. Obligation is unromantic at its very best, so unless you can lie back and think of England, just skip the whole thing. Until you're okay, forget it.

"Find other ways to be intimate" is other advice you'll hear. We all know what that means, and it doesn't mean cuddling, and frankly, I'd rather have sex and get something out of it than "find another way to be intimate." My husband feels differently and bravely offered himself up to these "other ways," the fooker.

I had a major improvement in health after surgery. I felt better than I had in years. This was therefore a time of renewed interest, to put it politely. Also, when I took the big dose of steroids that you take before certain kinds of chemo, I would lie there all night waking my husband up accidentally on purpose. "I'm sorry I woke you up, Honey. Since you're up anyway... ." If you ask my husband the biggest impact from this period, he will say that he believes in God now, because "God answered his most important and most fervent prayer."

I suggested that next time he might move "negative biopsy" up the list a notch.

But until you're okay, forget it. It's just like high school: if they love you, they'll wait. And I heard that from Dear Abby.

SHOULD A BREAST BE SUCH A BIG DEAL?

I started cancer treatment with what I thought was a feminist view of my breast. It is a body part, I said, like an elbow. I have finished using it for its function, which is feeding babies and not just entertaining troops, so it shouldn't be missed, kind of like an appendix or tonsils. I thought I was a little weird, because so many women fear breast cancer more than anything, yet the idea never occurred to me even when I went for my mammograms. So I figured that I would breeze through the mastectomy thing, and I pretty much did, emotionally.

I was ready to have perky breasts and kind of excited about it. And my new reconstructed breast is just beautiful. Nonetheless, at some point you're going to have to face the sexual fact that it looks like a breast but isn't quite exactly one. You're not going to have the same wonderful sensations that you had in the past. You can enjoy different ones, but not the same.

When I first started "getting to know" my new breast, I thought it was cool to have this new sensation that felt like a back rub on your breast. I did tricks with my new breast, since it is still connected to a back muscle, but absolutely nobody thought this was funny except me. Most people, including my best friend and my surgeon, two of the grossest people I know, said "Stop that." I tried it on a wide range of people, too. Anyway, pretty soon I felt that my "normal" breast should be the focus of sexuality, and it definitely gets more attention than my reconstructed one.

I couldn't help but think about what makes the breast so important. Am I a man trapped in a woman's body, I thought, given how much time I spent thinking about this? Anyway, here's what I came up with.

I think I can now argue that it is the breast, not the brain or the soul, which separates humans from animals. I know that sounds nuts. Usually people say that it is laughter, reason, mathematics, love, charity, language, a smile, or even killing a creature without needing it for food.

But any hyena can laugh, and it is the ugliest and awfulest animal on earth, any horse trying to unseat a rider seems to have reason, any dog knows enough math to know if you have given him his two treats or not. Love? Many species mate for life. Charity? Elephants help each other. Language? Study a bee dance. A smile? Oh please, the chimpanzee puts us to shame. Killing for the heck of it? You've never had a cat?

Humans, however, are the only species who show their mammary glands fully inflated even when they are not lactating. We are the only species I know of in which mammary glands cause arousal in both genders. Have I ruined the romance for you yet? My point is, breasts have an integral physical function in our lives as human mammals or they wouldn't be so prominent. The penis, though, only advertises itself when it wants to, even though the information when it does so could be quite helpful to the prospective and discerning mate.

So, it's not just "society" that makes you feel weird about losing a breast, and it's not just "not feeling maternal" and it's not just "male domination." You're a mammal who was designed this way for some reason. Your new body is going to take some getting used to, even if you love it. I don't own a single bra now, which is the morning prayer I say every day. "Thank you, God, for giving me cancer so that bras are a thing of the past." If you are a big-breasted woman, you know that this seems like kind of a fair trade. But it still takes some time.

I don't know why God or evolution or both designed us this way, but I do have a theory if it was God.

Since God created the universe eons ago, we can safely assume that He was in fact a teenager at the time. What does this mean and how can I prove it?

Have you ever watched those baboons with the big red bottoms, presumably made by our mutual Creator? They greet each other by turning around *and putting the big red bottom in someone else's face.* The other baboons don't scream, smack the red bottom or run away. They look at it for a long time, nice and closely, and then *eat a bug off of it.*

Spend an hour with a group of teenage boys and my theory will begin to make sense. Who else would think of the big red bottom except a teenage boy? Who else could invent the burp? And who is more obsessed with breasts than a teenage boy? Scientists have long known that if you write the Gettysburg Address on a poster of a topless woman, the average American boy will still be able to recite it 40 years later, and we now know that this is the only known way to remember the Periodic Table of the Elements. If you don't believe me, just watch Jeopardy, where the men *always* know their Table and the women just hardly ever do.

It's not a real big step from giving someone a big red ass to giving someone breasts that stay out all the time. I feel confident that a scientific writer could really sink his teeth into this topic and enlighten us all. I should write the theory down on a nice photograph of myself and send one a note.

WHAT DOES MODESTY MEAN AGAIN?

If you've already had a medical experience in which the whole world has seen your innards, like childbirth or really extensive dental work, you may not care about just how many people will be looking at your body and usually touching it, too.

On the other hand, you may still prefer to keep your body to yourself. You may need to do a little communicating with the medical teams to have things be the way you need. Nowadays, a lot of doctors are sensitive about modesty and privacy and will tell you before they touch anything or even look at anything. I am glad, but given that my modesty index is below zero, sometimes it just seems like really, really bureaucratic sex. "I am going to move your johnny off your shoulder. I am going to look at your breast. I am going to touch your breast."

If you are having trouble with the whole modesty problem, be sure to tell everybody that. Your feelings may change about this and you may be more or less sensitive about it as you go along, and you may feel differently after surgery than before. I always felt that it was my own decision to check my modesty at the door, not the doctor's, and I never had anyone violate that feeling.

Of course, my own solution was to establish a new policy: If I had to be topless for an appointment, *everybody* did. Everyone would laugh and I would have to tear the shirts off a resident or two before they knew I meant it.

We all hate those hospital gowns, right? At the Radiation department, you go to a changing room, change in to a johnny, then sit in the waiting area with everyone. On the radiation table you take the johnny off anyway, so I'm thinking that I can save myself some time if I don't change at all. I tell Ingrid and Rachel, the radiation therapists, that I'm not modest. I'll come into the room in my clothes, pull my top off, and get on the table, skipping the whole changing room thing. They gently explain the good reasons why the system works well the way it is, but they are responsive to my needs and off I go.

I'm feeling confident, a take charge kind of gal, one who strides topless like Hippolyta, queen of the Amazons, and fears nothing. God laughs but I don't hear it.

The next day I check in, skip the changing room, go to the radiation room striding like a biker chick and zip off my top. I turn around to greet Ingrid and Rachel.

Hmmm. I would appear to be in the wrong room, because Ingrid and Rachel are not there. Tom, Jeff and Robert look very surprised.

Ah, modesty.

Too Darn Hot: Menopause and Chemotherapy

IF YOU ARE GETTING NEAR MENOPAUSE, chemo will probably push you into it. When I first experienced this, life was easy.

THE INNOCENT ME WROTE THIS:

Chemotherapy can push you into menopause; this may mean a few symptoms. I learned something from *Woman to Woman*: "Although there has been a great deal of attention directed to the experience of passing through menopause, you may find, as many of us did, that when you are coping with cancer, menopause pales in comparison; it is simply not that big a deal."

A LITTLE LATER IT WASN'T SO EASY. I WROTE THIS:

I did have "some symptoms." I bought a miracle product called Astroglide, which may be the most embarrassing product name I've ever bought. It has a vaguely Jetsons sound to it but not in a good way. It's a product for "personal intimate dryness." It turns out to have so many lubricating uses that you will wonder how you ever did without it. It's the baking soda of sex! If you were Heloise, you would be writing books and books of helpful hints.

My hot flashes picked up the pace in the summer while I was recover-

141 • TOO DARN HOT: MENOPAUSE AND CHEMOTHERAPY

ing from surgery. I learned to keep a fan on, very low, aimed just near my face but not directly at it. This would keep me comfortable all night. It reminded me of sleeping outside at the beach, when you get this incredible breeze on your cheeks. So you turn on the fan and you can fall asleep imagining the sounds that go along with sleeping on the beach, which in my case is my husband's voice, *"Do you know how much we are spending renting this house and you want to sleep* OUTSIDE?"

As winter came, I enjoyed my hot flashes more. I started wearing moisturizer with sunscreen in it, not only because the dermatologist wants you to, but because I loved the smell of being on vacation at the beach whenever I had a hot flash, which was so often that life was one long August.

I noticed that I was going tropical in many ways. I ditched the heavy, timeworn, dark and beautiful mahogany tables in our bedroom and replaced them with rickety bamboo cabinets. "I see we moved to Florida," my husband said when we went to bed that night. I was humming a Beach Boys song at the time and didn't hear him. Lucky for him I don't get mood swings, isn't it?

If your tumor is estrogen receptive (ask your oncologist) then you won't be able to seek relief in hormone therapy or natural sources of estrogen. But doctors have remedies for hot flashes and other symptoms, so as always *be sure to call.*

Lots of people say that their skin gets drier in menopause and in chemotherapy. I attacked this from the beginning, as I already had dry and sensitive skin and didn't want more. I read lots of advice, which all said "Use a rich moisturizer." Oh for heaven's sake, what does that mean? Is there some law that you can't tell someone what you use? Other people will tell you that it doesn't matter what you use, that it's all hype, that you just need a bar of soap. And size doesn't matter either.

So here's what I used. I tried a lot of stuff and narrowed it down to these. For my face, a gentle cleanser: I liked Physician's Advice, their cleanser called Gentle. This brand is available at the web site hsn.com. In the summer, I used Bobbi Brown's Intensive Moisturizer. Bobbi Brown is a department store brand. It doesn't have sunscreen in it as of this writing, and you may be able to get away with a lighter formula anyway during the summer, but I couldn't. In the winter, I used Physician's Advice Intensive Oil-Free Moisturizer – not the gentle, the Intensive. I used these morning and night. None of this works that well if you don't exfoliate. If your skin is very sensitive from chemotherapy, which sometimes happens, then skip the exfoliating or do it very gently. I liked Bobbi Brown's exfoliant because it didn't strip my skin.

On my body, I used Lac-Hydrin Five, which is a drugstore brand. For a few days after chemotherapy it would sometimes be a little too strong and my skin would redden where I put it. Being Irish, I have that skin that reddens all the time anyway, so it wasn't a big deal. If you prefer something fancier or creamier, use it on top of the Lac-Hydrin. Lac-Hydrin worked because it actually penetrated my non-face hide, and nothing else seemed to. I am made like a cheap vinyl pocket book, and it takes some power to get through that.

For some reason, after chemotherapy was completed, my skin could tolerate more products than it could before. I discovered a major addiction to skin care. I started buying kits from Signature Club A and Serious Skin Care, using Cellex-C, Oil of Olay with SPF and L'Occitane shea butter hand cream. None of these products are inexpensive. But given how much money I've wasted over the years, I was just relieved to find things that worked for me. If other companies believe that their product is better, I would be more than happy to try some free samples. I can probably be bought for the right lipstick.

There are also classes in many cities that can help you with make-up tips and all that. Your oncology department can probably tell you about them. There wasn't one available around when I needed it, but everybody who goes says they are fun and you get great free stuff. Check out websites cancerandcareers.org and lookgoodfeelbetter.org for information.

A YEAR LATER, WHEN I FOUND OUT THAT ALL I HAD HAD SO FAR WAS BABY MENOPAUSE, I WROTE THIS:

Holy Crap.

I still use moisturizer out of sheer optimism, that I won't sweat it off before I make it out the front door. I go out the front door out of optimism too – will today be the day I find the car keys? Will it be the day I remember where I dropped the kids off?

And then, worst of all, I found out that we women do menopause just like we do pregnancy, childbirth and going to the ladies room: we like to do it together. In groups. We like everyone to do it the same way and we can tell if you belong in our club or not by how you do it. And so, I found that menopause advice sounded exactly like, you guessed it, cancer advice, pregnancy advice, you name it.

The first hundred or so times I've learned this, I've been able to smile at our foibles, but now I was so impossibly sick of it I could scream, so I did, just like I did when I found out that breathing doesn't actually relieve pain in childbirth, it just gives you something to keep you busy. The more research I did, I became just a tad dispirited, mean and bitter, like the dried herbs I was supposed to eat without water, which might dilute its healing chi or something. Want to send your healer into a little tizzy? Bring a cup of coffee with you and wash your herbs down with it.

As usual, it would turn out that life had something to teach me. But first, I took my usual first step of making bitter fun of everybody else. I started with the many clubs of menopause.

There's the Goddess club, which is where you find women with naturally curly hair and long dresses and sandals doing something with a maypole without recognizing that maypoles look a bit, well, familiar to the trained eye.

There's the Dorian Grey, or Joan Collins, club of menopause. This woman has her hair done every week and looks fabulous. She looks younger than the girls at the maypole but is not nearly as much fun. This is a woman who says that she never had any "of these silly issues" about staying home and being a homemaker. Her best friend remarks on the lime rickeys they had together most afternoons with the babysitter.

There's the Crone club. She also has naturally curly hair. She believes in the beautiful wisdom of women in menopause. She celebrates her wrinkles and even makes Raku pottery shapes out of them to give to her friends on their birthdays. She did a copper etching of her own vagina, which hangs in the kitchen. She used 100% cotton tampons and laundered them and then passed them on to her teenagers, who "lost" them.

There's the Stoic club. If you never ever knew when she had her period even though you shared an office, she thinks you'll never know she's in menopause. She is undeniably a strong person, but it has been two years since her last smile and absolutely, positively, under no circumstances should you ever let her be in charge of office birthday parties, because she only makes non-fat soy cakes with carob frosting dusted with flax.

Then there's the Role Model club. She is active, exercising nearly every day. She and her partner eat a healthy diet. She laughs about hot flashes, with a silvery laugh. She rides her bike on vacation with her grandchildren, whom she calls "grandbabies." In a movie she would be played by Doris Day. I love her.

Next is the Post Office club of Menopause: a woman who looks like she just shot somebody, somebody who deserved it real bad. She sure as hell didn't get her hair done this week and the last time someone called her a crone she took out her bullwhip. In the other pocket of her holster, there is a bottle of whiskey. She wears that T-shirt that says "I am out of estrogen and I have a gun," but she does not belong to the NRA, only because she thinks they are a bunch of liberal pansies.

I found that quite a few websites use the words "wimmin, wymin or womon." When I was younger this was very important to me, until I realized that I like to use words like "tramp" instead. I wanted to feel it was still important to use the words, because it is. I just couldn't stand the inevitable link between feminism and soy.

Still. I kept doing research. I found that there is enormous money ready to be made in the baby boomer's menopause. People everywhere are looking for non-hormone cures for hot flashes as busily as we once looked for

Scandinavian baby carriages. This is good news, because money follows the baby boomer into every thing she wants, and then we move on and leave the world a marginally improved place. Head out to the baby store today and see how much we improved the convenience of taking care of a baby. First there were the plastic bottle liners – great, but you had to stretch them over the lip of the bottle. We bequeath a major improvement there: you just drop in a plastic, honest-to-God, condom. The manufacturer believes that the woman using this product does not recognize it, probably true.

TAMOXIFEN, FEMARA, ARIMIDEX

If you are taking one of these cousins and have few side effects, you are among the many. Skip this section, because you won't learn a thing. If you are having a symptom or two or eleven, read on.

When I finished most of this book I had just started taking tamoxifen. If your cancer is estrogen receptive, you'll be taking it too, or something like it. You won't be taking any hormone replacement therapy, because tamoxifen and other drugs work by trying to keep your cancer cells from getting any estrogen.

There are two categories of drugs that you may be given to prevent recurrences. Both are diets for your cancer cells, depriving them of estrogen as if it were carbs. The tamoxifen type works on keeping the estrogen your body produces from reaching any cancer cells that may remain. You can take it whether you are pre- or post- menopausal.

The second type is aromatase inhibitors. After your ovaries give up, your body still produces estrogen. Your adrenal gland produces an enzyme that converts testosterone to estrogen – guess where? In your FAT. Just think of all those little male hormones being turned into female ones, starting life over in a fat cell. I don't know exactly why this makes me laugh – it's the idea of millions of little men sucked into fat cells and, oops! I'm a woman now and I'm fat!

The aromatase inhibitors, like arimidex and femara, work by shutting that down. You can only take these if you are post-menopausal.

Many women who have never had cancer take these drugs if they have risk factors. They don't guarantee no cancer, but they reduce your chances of getting it, like taking an umbrella to keep it from raining.

Many people get no side effects from these drugs, and I was confident that I would be fine. I was, for months. So, of course, having sprinted across the treatment finish line, I tripped two feet later.

I had already experienced chemotherapy-induced menopause, temporarily as it turned out. I thought it was pretty easy to cope with. What I didn't know is that tamoxifen pills love to hear women say that menopause isn't so bad. They sit on the shelf eavesdropping at the pharmacy, and they write your name down. "We'll show YOU," they laugh. They will take you on a nostalgic trip in which normal menopause symptoms will seem like a summer breeze. They could design an amusement park ride based on these symptoms and even the teenagers would be begging to get off.

If you are going to get side effects from tamoxifen, you may have them in the beginning and find that they go away. Mine started months after I started taking it. Intense and constant hot flashes, tens and tens of them every day and night. Fatigue. Insomnia. Light-headedness. Forgetfulness. Tendency to depression. Tendency to dehydration despite constant drinking, which leads to heart skipping. I could not find any time in a day when I did not feel miserable, for weeks on end.

Worst of all, the forgetfulness centered on my wallet. I lost three wallets in one month, with plenty of cash in each one. Whoever found them and didn't return them, I hope you read this and feel like smacking yourself, which you should go ahead and do right now. Do you know how much time I have spent renewing licenses alone? The lady at the Registry says, friendly-like, "See you soon!"

Best of all? Tamoxifen gives you the symptoms of menopause, but not menopause itself, another one of those hilarious cancer ironies. So, while you deal with all of this, you can get periods too. Cramps and hot flashes at the same time? This, I realized on a bad day, is why gun control is so, so important.

Many people get no symptoms and no periods. I wanted to write about this in case you are not so lucky, and also because I learned a lot by finding out that cancer really had not turned me into any kind of hero. I was quickly and firmly back in Chicken Land.

To begin with, villains everywhere use sleep deprivation to torture people. If you've had a newborn in the house, or a kid with chronic ear infections, you know what I mean. The sleep deprivation intensified everything. Remember the Vince Lombardi idea that fatigue makes cowards of us all? Let's just say I was really, really fatigued.

So, during the sleep deprivation I began to lose the perspective I had about my new body. I became much more focused on the mastectomy. I had more pain throughout the area. I felt frustrated that I would have to live with this new body forever. Little things about it bothered me – like when you have an itch on your back and it takes awhile to find a spot that will relieve it because of the nerves being disconnected. I lost any patience for any one else's problems except those of my closest friends and family.

I even – though I know my husband would say this isn't so — became just a teeny, weeny bit more easily irritated than usual. When you combine this with selfishness, it can be just a tad hard to deal with — for which I would like to apologize to the elderly woman in front of me at the super market, for asking why she would bother living so long if she is going to spend her life whining, and are those expired coupons older than she is or are they just older than dirt?

Worst of all, I had written this stupid book. Courage? Not exactly. I spent my mornings whining; in the afternoon I would upgrade to complaining. Each evening was spent moaning. Throughout the night, I would sigh heavily to make sure that nobody else could sleep either. Even my best friend asked me if I thought it was a good idea to write this book when I wasn't displaying any actual courage of any kind.

My doctors were great and they offered a number of solutions which are often effective, but they didn't work for me. I even thought that maybe I would stop taking tamoxifen but not tell anyone that I had done so. I know this sounds awful, but I could not stand it another minute and yet I did not want to worry anybody.

After weeks of whining I even tried some sleeping pills, to get some relief. While the side effects continued to get worse, getting some sleep greatly increased my ability to cope. However, I reached a point in which I still felt that I was damned if my life was going to be something I "cope" with. If I deeply enjoyed my life through hell and high water in the past, why couldn't I do that now?

I realized that because of the sleep deprivation I had not gotten my mind around the problem. I had to go back to the beginning and go through the same damn steps that I had taken through treatment. I started by asking if this were the worst thing that ever happened to me. I spent a moment feeling grateful that it was not. Then I started out trying to awaken the courage muscle all over again.

As I started through the steps again, I began to feel a whole lot better and a whole lot happier, which made me feel more hopeful. Then, of course, my hot flashes got ... worse. I headed down the spiral again.

I think I tried everything. Effexor, clonidine, catapres patch, neurontin, megace, tibolone, Vitamin E, paced breathing, layered dressing, bellergal, air conditioning, showers, fans, cold compresses, and acupuncture. Even though I once lived in Hong Kong, I was fairly skeptical about acupuncture. "Fairly skeptical" is Chinese for "I think it is really stupid." It turned out to feel wonderful, and I highly recommend it, even though it did not cure my hot flashes.

Eventually, I stopped taking tamoxifen. From the intense sweating, I became severely dehydrated and developed parotitis, an infection of the salivary gland, that, ironically, can be spelled using the letters from the expression "pair o' tits." I was in the hospital for a week, but that's not what bothered me. You know how every August there will be a county fair somewhere and they find the world's biggest hog? That's exactly what I looked like from the parotitis. I told the doctors that's what I looked like and they all seriously shook their heads no. Then I heard them out in the hall and they were actually crying from laughing so hard.

I tried arimidex and femara, both just as bad. It is not a popular decision to stop taking these drugs, but for me it had become a major quality of life issue. The extra safety of taking these drugs was not as great as the burden, unlike actual treatment.

The worst news about this whole mess? Unfortunately, just like in every other damn problem you'll ever have, one of the best medicines is exercise. I had fallen off the exercise wagon during radiation and had only made half-hearted attempts to get back on. I started exercising again after I started acupuncture, and of course it helped somewhat. This reminded me again that I have major disagreements with how this universe is organized.

If I were to end this section with the meaningful inspirational quote that I reflected on during this period, it would be: "Screw this." I felt better during many days of chemotherapy than I did now. I refused to be called a "cancer survivor." I wanted to be called a "long suffering cancer victim" instead.

If you think all the advice you got after your diagnosis was irritating, just wait until you start complaining about your hot flashes and other symptoms. Everybody copes with it better than you do. It's only American women who suffer, you know. Asian women don't. American women are nuts and eat too much. You need to eat soy. You need herbs. You need to meditate. You need to think positively, that's what you need. You need to worship a goddess. You need incense. You need to stop using soap and deodorant. You are a victim of male dominance. You are resisting your croning, you need to celebrate being a wise goddess. You shouldn't eat meat. You need to try this herb – I know it's estrogen, but it's natural! You're going about this all the wrong way and you need to go to this health place in Western Massachusetts.

At this point I started listening – did someone just say they're taking me to Canyon Ranch? A spa? Facials? Body scrubs? Of course not. This health place turned out to be a yoga camp for people who wish to live a simpler life, which is Buddhist for "Bring Your Own Sheets." Turns out that it's the owners who want a simpler life, who want their chi flowing freely, uncluttered by laundry or decorating or mattresses. Turns out you sleep in bunk beds, which I have not been able to do since the 100 years of torture I endured at the hands of my most evil sister. Still makes me twitch.

After a year and a half of nearly constant hot flashes, I feel deeply challenged by this. Your oncologist may not give you estrogen if your tumor is estrogen receptive. Some will, some won't. And you learn that no matter who your doctors are, your oncologist is driving the bus. He or she trumps everybody else. Try asking your gynecologist for some estrogen. "Sure," you'll hear. "Just let me check with Oncology." Great — the check's in the mail, my e-mail wasn't working, I'll still respect you in the morning, and now, "Let me check with Oncology."

I began to rethink my view of the saintly Oncologist. I was wrong, I realized — they are actually evil, power hungry demons who got pushed around in medical school by those orthopedic guys who were constantly playing basketball with George Clooney. They made a vow, sealed in blood not their own, to be in charge of every decision those other doctors would ever make.

I did figure out a way to get some hormones, though. My plan: you know that little stash of Percocet you saved after surgery or childbirth or whatever? Take it to the next PTO meeting. Announce that you have some and offer to trade it for estrogen. The next sound you hear will be 25 pocketbooks flipping open and you'll just name your price.

I tried a drug called tibolone, which is currently not available in the U.S., so of course it is easy to get online. It is not FDA approved, it's not yet recommended for cancer patients, but I read a lot about it and decided to try it. No luck, but tibolone has been used in Europe for years to control menopause symptoms. It is a created steroid, not an estrogen, but it has properties of estrogen, progestin and androgen.

I have accepted that the only road out of this is a mental one. I am trying to view each hot flash as a single incident, like a stubbed toe, and not a cumulative problem. This is hard to do when your sweat is dripping so much that people can hear it and your husband keeps getting up to check the faucets. I also turn bright red, as if I'm not pink enough already. People will gape at me and ask if I am okay. If I like them I explain, if I don't I tell them I must have forgotten to take my antibiotics and they might want to consult a health care professional.

I call this the Tower of Terror method. Because I am such a chicken, I have had to develop a mental approach in which I promise to be scared when something is actually scary, but not scared when it isn't. So I can stand on line for a ride with the kids, and be okay. I always ask how long the ride is, and then I plan to be terrified for that long. And I get truly terrified, but I confine it to the moment.

I am trying this with hot flashes. I am aware of a hot flash when it happens and then I move on, instead of staying imprisoned by dreading the next one. If I had been able to do this in labor maybe I wouldn't have needed all that ether.

If chemo pushes you into menopause, I hope it is easy for you. The good news is that since people have become afraid of hormone replacement therapy, the race is on for drug companies to find other methods. I hope they find one that I can take until it turns out to be harmful.

Be careful to review everything you try with your doctor, and especially check in before you take any herbs or supplements. There is some terrible advice out there. One particularly dangerous web site actually recommends giving up chocolate to ease menopause symptoms.

I don't have an ending to this story yet. I have to find a way to tolerate estrogen depletion.

AND THEN A LITTLE LATER I WROTE THIS:

One night I was sitting online dripping sweat onto the keyboard and I thought about the role of the hypothalamus. The hypothalamus is one of those things you never notice until you start getting older, just like your knees. It controls temperature and is part of the brain. On a whim, thinking about the brain, I typed in "hypnosis" and "hot flashes" into Google. One medical study came back, which is the first time I got fewer than four million results. Some physicians had studied using hypnosis on hot flashes in breast cancer patients.

I couldn't wait to see which Boston hospital had done the study. Hmm, Corner Brook. Hadn't heard of it, so it must be in New York. Hmmm. Kept looking.

Corner Brook is in Newfoundland, which I thought was technically at the very end of the earth. You may have thought that the poles are the ends of the earth, I would say, but no, because those are so much easier to get to.

So, of course it turns out that Newfoundland is easy to get to, beautiful and friendly. Its people are particularly individualistic, by which I mean that it is apparently considered boring for everyone to speak the same way at the same time. There are 500,000 people in Newfoundland but there are at least 600,000 different accents. My favorite was that of a young man who told me that he voted for the new premier because "he is a liar." I expressed surprise and asked him why. "He's very smart and went to school to learn how to be one," he said. "Where I come from, we're born liars," I said. "We don't need school for that." Our conversation went on like that for quite awhile until I figured out that he was saying "lawyer."

There are plenty of hypnotists in Boston, but I went to Newfoundland anyway. I was too desperate to wait for someone else to learn this specific treatment, when there was a doctor who had already tried it. So, my friend Laura and I got on what they used to call a "plane" before air travel was technically invented yet. My doctors were supportive.

The doctor in Newfoundland met us at the airport and took us home for dinner. We traveled to his house in the woods as darkness fell, crossing a one-lane bridge to a dirt road. As we crossed the bridge, my friend asked in a whisper if I knew this guy wasn't an axe murderer. No, I said, he might be, plus he looks kind of Scottish.

And so began one of the most interesting weeks of my life. We loved him, his family and his dog. They welcomed us, fed us, entertained us and made us laugh. His daughter told us that this doctor had the habit of stealing desserts from his children at the table. When caught, he would look surprised and say "I do apologize." The poor cake-less children believed his polite apology the first fifty or sixty times, but eventually learned cynicism and how to eat really fast and under the table with the dog, who was much less likely to steal food than their father was.

It does seem to me that a guy who knows hypnosis would be able to get as many desserts as he wanted, but I loved this phrase and I use it now whenever I do something mean on purpose.

I'm writing this when I've back home for two whole days. So does it work? Yes. It is a tool, not a cure, but it is powerful and I feel it will be very helpful. That's all I can say now, but I'm pretty excited.

And I also got to try curling, which is that Canadian sport that is actually very interesting but has a way of making people who play it look a little, well, drunk. One person shoves a 44-pound rock with a handle on it down an ice rink. The other people run in front of the rock, sweeping the ice to help make the rock go faster. You have a broom, and it really is a broom, and you sweep like crazy as if company is coming and the house smells of all the spilled cat litter.

A LITTLE WHILE LATER I WROTE THIS:

Ha-ha. After all this, I came out of menopause. Sound like good news? Not in the perverse world of oncology. Your chances of survival are better if you are post-menopausal, so oncologists like to put you there. If you remain pre-menopausal after treatment, you may have the same issue I did, so here's what I know.

Your ovaries need to be shut down. You can do that surgically or chemically. If you never want to have another pregnancy and feel you can tolerate the hormonal changes, surgery removes your ovaries, with the added benefit of preventing ovarian cancer.

The chemical approach is a monthly shot, in my case Lupron. I went online, read a few bulletin boards and saw that a lot of women hate these drugs and feel awful on them. There was very little information from women using it for cancer, most was about using a smaller dose to treat endometriosis.

As always, you have a choice. Do you believe that the enhanced survival chances are worth the burden? This time I thought yes. I went in for my first shot.

I woke up the next day to find that my feet were dangling over the jaws of hell. The hot flashes, impossibly, increased. I was given a nice case of instant depression, very deep. I desperately went back and read my own stupid book again. I worked on trying to find a way to live with this.

And then, miraculously wonderful, came the first relief I've felt in a long time. I woke up a few days after the shot feeling better than I had since my disaster with tamoxifen. My gynecologist's theory is that it was the roller coaster of being in and out of menopause that was bothering me, not the low estrogen itself. My body could never adjust. The way I feel now is exactly how I felt with chemo-induced menopause. I have hot flashes but it's not that bad most of the time. At this point, though, I've only had a month's worth. I'm optimistic.

Later, after two treatments, it seems that I will have an initial period of intense hot flashes and chemically-induced depression, then for a few days before the next shot I will start another little hormonal roller coaster. We decided to switch me to the three-month version of the shot, which is time-released, in order to have these transitions happen less often. I've had my first three-month shot and it's very different — a more gradual transition in, a little more feeling wired. I can tolerate this and expect to continue the shots for a few years.

What did I learn through this? Just as with cancer, find your own way through menopause. If you are in the Ageless club, you may not get estrogen but you'll still be out there with great hair and a facelift or two. Crone and Goddess? Dance away around that maypole. Stoic and Role Model? I want to be you in my next life and maybe I'll marry Rock Hudson when I grow up. Post Office? Come sit by me.

If you have gone through pregnancy, childbirth, adoption and cancer the way everyone wanted you to, then let menopause be the time you choose your own road. Try every club, be in a different one everyday, start your own.

Found A Peanut: The Last Chapter Turns Out To Be Chapter One

DO YOU KNOW THOSE AWFUL KIDS' SONGS that keep starting again? Over and over again, you think it's finished, and off the kids go again. They like to sing these in the car on long trips. When you leave the driveway, it feels so festive. Hours later, you and your husband are no longer speaking to each other after realizing who-forgot-to-bring-whatever. His lips are tightly drawn and he is staring at the highway ahead as if it were just another road to his doom. He is fantasizing that he is driving a Corvette and you are not the woman in the passenger seat. You are sitting absolutely silent except for your occasional hopeless sigh. And from the back seat, relentlessly, comes "Just now I found a peanut... ."

For many people, that's what cancer becomes. It's never over, because there will always be another check-up, another test, another biopsy. I've made up my mind to avoid the daily pain of that. I am still new to the cancer business, but if I don't do anything else, I will still try my best to end that

Henry Vaughn was one of those 17th century metaphysical poets like John Donne, who they keep reciting in that cancer play/movie Wit. But Vaughn was also a doctor. He wrote a lot of depressing stuff about being still alive while everyone else was dead, so, okay, maybe he wasn't that good of a doctor.

stupid song. Here's what I mean.

When I was nearing the end of chemotherapy, feeling like I was just the bravest and toughest person in the world, my brother-in-law e-mailed me a wake-up call. Rick is an oncologist and he sent me an article by Hester Hill Schnipper at Beth Israel Deaconess Medical Center in Boston, where I was being treated. She is the head of social work for Oncology. Guess what I learned as I was almost finished with treatment? More women seek help – counseling, support groups – *after* treatment than during it.

Great. Just when it was over.

I remember getting a call from Hester early on, offering help, and I told her that I was okay, but thanks. She said that sometimes women like to come in for a support group when they have finished treatment. Okay, I said, thinking that was golldurn unlikely, but thanks.

You would think that I would have learned by now that when I say I don't need help, God will find some charming way to remind me that I do. It turns out that the surgeons and oncologists can remove the cancer but they can't remove the fear. Is it going to come back? Is that freckle the same or does it now look suspicious? Is that a new lump? Am I going to spend the rest of my life looking for lumps and checking my freckles? And, above all, God forbid, am I ever going to have to live through treatment *again*? Because, God, I know for absolutely, positively sure that I can't do that.

I thought the song was almost over, but now here we went with another verse. Then I got the chance to test drive life after cancer, even before treatment was over. I found a brand new lump. To avoid any suspense, I'll skip to the end first and tell you that it was totally fine and nothing to worry about.

In the meantime, I'd had my wake-up call and decided that this really was a test drive. How would I handle it?

At some point I figured out that I probably have about 16,000 days remaining in my life, which I decide are like money. If I know that I only have $16,000 that has to last me for the rest of my life, am I going to spend two, or three, or any of those dollars on worrying? I've met so many people who suffer through every biopsy of their lives, who even worry until they get their Pap test results every year. I think for some people that's the best way to deal with it. But for me, I don't want to spend any of my "time dollars" on worry. So I go about my normal life and feel great that I can. I make sure that I am going to be very busy for a couple of days, because when I need to keep my mind off of something that's the only legal thing that works.

I also think about the people I've known who have died before their time. They had no warnings and no guarantees of living to be 90, because nobody has. Now that we know that a friend died at 50, do we think he should have spent his last years worrying about it?

To me, when you finish treatment, you can start with a clean slate. Your chances of cancer may be a little higher than someone else's – but on the other hand, you're going to be getting a lot more tests than most people, so at least you'll know.

At this point I heard something helpful from my sister-in-law. She had cancer, and she also had a neighbor who was a Holocaust survivor. The neighbor came to ask her if her treatment was done. Laura said yes. The neighbor said, "Good. Now, FORGET about it." These are powerful words.

So I had the biopsy and honestly and truly put it out of mind. Two days later, the phone rings and I get the report that it's nothing. I let my husband know pretty casually. His sigh of relief breaks my heart. Were you really worried, I ask him. Quit it, he says, and I do. The next day, at my father's 84th birthday, everyone asks me how I am. I say great and mention the biopsy. Then I realize that every single person already knows about it, because everybody called everybody.

I remembered again that you don't have cancer alone. I am still trying to figure out how to help your husband, wife, friend, relative, child, parent cope with their lives during treatment and after it ends. I don't have any answers, but I'm seriously considering keeping all biopsies to myself. Since I don't worry, why make anyone else worry? This is probably not a good idea.

There would be other lumps and other biopsies in the future. I thought I would treat these as I had the first one, that I wouldn't waste any time worrying about it. Ha!

I found another new lump in my breast on a Friday night, when I wouldn't be able to do anything constructive about it for a few days. I tried using it as a little worry bead, but that proved to be kind of gross plus the other people in church complained.

So here I was. I had made fun of people who called any old lump a "brush with cancer." I had breezed through biopsies, even the cancerous one, with nary a worry. I was totally prepared to face a lifetime of occasional worry without losing any sleep. Now ... I was, well, panicked.

I told my sister. Turns out that Terri doesn't believe in wasting any time worrying either, at least, not about me. Terri developed a unique approach. She urged me never to tell family or friends again when I found a lump. Instead, she sent me a "phone tree" she developed just for this occasion. I would start with the first person on the list, move on to the next, etc.

The first person on the list would be Customer Service at WalMart. I was to get on line for Returns. The clerk would be so grateful that I had nothing to return that he or she would be happy to hear about my lump, unlike, say, my sister Terri. I would move on to calling AOL customer service, which would give me the same result plus I would use up a lot of worry time sitting on hold. If that didn't get me through the weekend, I should go to the airport and be sure to be searched. They would find the lump and x-ray me right away. End of worry, no need to tell the family.

I then understood that commercial in which the woman is on the phone actually crying to her pharmacist that she has breast cancer and the pharmacist actually has all the time in the world. I thought this was hysterical when I first saw it. I pictured the phone options at the typical pharmacy: "To cry, press 2. Begin crying at the tone." But in Terri's model, the pharmacist is the perfect person to call. You just became a profitable customer, so the pharmacist cares, unlike, say, my sister Terri.

Michael was out of town. Fortunately, I have other sisters. Colette and her partner Laura actually spent the day with me, took me for the doctor's appointment. We had fun.

It may be that worrying about each check-up or each biopsy is just your way of handling things. If you are otherwise functioning, fine. Bob Champion, the jockey who won the world's most grueling horse race after cancer, says that "every January I return to The Royal Marsden Hospital in Sutton for a check-up. I don't sleep for at least the week before, because I am still so terrified. I can smell the chemotherapy as soon as I turn off the (highway) M25, and I am still six miles away from the hospital." (His book "*Champion's Story*" tells the whole tale.) Anyway, this is a man who functioned fully after cancer, to say the least. Setting up a Cancer Trust, opening two clinics, running a business, being a motivational speaker. If he wants to lose sleep for a week, I say fine, and if you want to do the same, I say fine too. The goal is that someday worrying will be a part-time job, not a full-time one.

But if it's really keeping you awake, I recommend calling my sister Terri, day or night. She's in the book.

WHERE DID ALL THE CASSEROLES GO?

Onto the next big problem of the end of treatment: you're not going to be the center of attention anymore. I know that's a very harsh way to say it.

Many people talk about their family and friends wanting to feel that the cancer is over when the treatment ends, but the patient feels deserted by this and wants the family to be sensitive. As for me, I think the family and friends have been through enough, and that they *should* feel this way. Maybe now it's *their* turn to be taken care of a little. So as soon as you're feeling better, however long that takes, *let* them feel it's over. They deserve the break. As patients, we deserve the little kick in the pants this gives us. It hurts a bit, or a lot, but it's a good quick way back to normal life.

This is hard, because for months we have been so cared for. Yes, we've suffered. But most of us, thankfully, have someone who picks up the reins sometimes along the way. It's time to share the work again. But who wants to?

It reminds me of your second pregnancy. In your first, your husband carries you gently to the couch on hearing the news, showers you with gentle kisses and peels you grapes until the delivery. In your second, well, maybe he'll clean the older one's barf off the couch if you're really sick, but there's no lying down on that couch, is there? So, in a way, you miss that first pregnancy, even if it was hard. I think the transition out of treatment is the same. It's like coming out of a dark cave. You wanted to come out, you were dying to, but now that sun sure hurts your eyes.

As much as I believe in letting everybody move on from focusing on you and your cancer, it's also true that the physical recovery from treatment takes a while, so don't give up that special treatment too soon. Tell everyone that "my treatment is finished, and I can't wait to feel all better. The doctor says it will take anywhere up to a few months, and I'm really looking forward to that." It reminds me of great advice I got from a nurse when my first baby was born. "Stay in a bathrobe for two weeks," she said. "Nobody will ask you to do anything." This really works. "Can I get you some coffee?" you say weakly. "No, no, no," your lazy ass aunt says, "what can I get *you*?"

Aaaaah, another coping strategy.

CAN I BUY A CORVETTE NOW?
(HAVE A LITTLE MID-LIFE CRISIS WITH YOUR CANCER)

Whether it's the early menopause caused by chemotherapy, or a life change caused by cancer, I don't know. I just know that by the end of treatment I was asking all those pesky questions that can keep you awake at night if you let them. Was the path I chose the one I was supposed to take in life? Have I made any contribution at all? Should I have kept pushing at my career? Should I start a new career now? Am I doing the right job for my kids? My husband? In my opinion cancer should give you a break from all this but it just got worse.

I haven't decided what to do with this yet, because the one thing I've always known is that you don't make big decisions when you are really tired. My decision and my advice to anyone who might experience this is to let this go a little bit until you're feeling really strong and don't need so much energy to devote to cancer. Otherwise, you'll consider the kind of choices I thought about, like becoming a Philanthropic Exotic Dancer for all of the undeserving poor who otherwise cannot afford a really good stripper, since I had these great new breasts and all. Gladly, my husband asked me "don't you have to know how to dance to do that?"

You already know that striving is life-giving, so I'm not telling you to go to sleep and forget about all this. Just that you don't have to do everything at once, and maybe your body and your mind are a little busy right now.

How bad did it get for me? I actually reached the point of feeling so mature that maybe it was time to *get rid of all of my pre-childbearing shoes*. All those adorable single-digit-size little things with the heels, that belong in the attic until after you die, when your kids wonder who on earth ever wore them. I hope they give them to their kids to play dress-up with because they are almost all dressy shoes that deserve a second life. They belong on a little girl who is also wearing an old prom dress, her mother's best lipstick and a tiara. And when a woman, or a very fashionable man, starts talking about giving them away, she is either ready to die or is totally out of storage space.

So now everyone knows why it was that with everything else going on in our crazy cancer-treatment lives, I decided to disrupt the house by adding more storage to the attic.

One of the great things about having cancer is that unlike most of your life, this calls on everything you've got. Your emotional, physical, mental, spiritual, social and intellectual strengths will be tested. To be honest, now that I'm done with treatment, I realize that I loved that part of it. I felt fully alive, because I had to. If I list the very happiest moments of my life, many are times when I felt that every part of me was called upon. This was one of them. Okay, the other times that called on everything wouldn't have killed me in time, but still.

Treatment was, in an odd way, like living in a long beer commercial, where everybody is going for the gusto, every minute counts, and there's throwing up involved. When life goes back to normal, your mind thinks it can stop living like that. For a while I started to feel bored, which is just one step from depression, then I finally realized what was going on. As Nietzsche wrote, "I have often asked myself whether I am not more heavily obligated to the hardest years of my life than to any others." I don't want to go too far down that Nietzsche road, because I keep trying to picture him in a support group and I don't think he'd be the best-loved member. A tad too depressing, I think. But I agree with him in the sense that crisis is kind of exhilarating.

So now I'm back to normal life, in which parts of me are still called upon – but none of these parts are things that I am actually good at. Just as I know that working full time at most jobs is easier than being home with kids, being in cancer treatment is emotionally easier than finishing it. It doesn't make sense, but it's true anyway.

I finally decided that I just have to find a few more things that call on me in this way. I don't know what they will all be yet. I mentioned to Michael that I'm thinking of taking a few college science courses, but the challenge would be that this time I would actually go to class. Also I would date less.

In the meantime, I got to know that woman with the whiskey and the whip, I kind of like her, and I hope she visits often.

YOU ARE WHAT YOU THINK ABOUT

On this day I am just about at the end of treatment. I am busy with my new hobby, which is sitting around feeling sorry for myself. Nobody Else Has Cancer. Nobody Else Has Trouble At Work. Nobody Else has a Messy House. Nobody Else Doesn't Know What to Do With Their Lives. Oh, and Nobody Loves Me.

I think about a new business idea of putting together those craft kits, only instead of "Gold Leaf Your Closet" kits it will be "The Complete Self-Pity Kit: Everything You Need for Feeling Sorry for Yourself." I'm unclear on what will be in it because I can't picture anything but chocolate. It will also have a recording of the Picard Boys, of my friend Laura's family, singing their rendition of the Beach Boys' "I Get Around," which is: Round, Round, Sit Around, I Sit Around, Round Round, ooh-ooh-ooh-oooh, I Sit Arouououououound.

I catch a glimpse of myself in the television screen as I flip between home shopping, infomercials and Martha Stewart. The attentive reader knows that Martha is a good mental health break, because you can feel so sane compared to this wonderful woman. It doesn't work today.

Anyway, I look awful. I look not only bored, but boring, and I see a few lines in my face. I'm feeling too lazy to remind myself that this feeling is usually just fatigue, when I hear music coming from downstairs. It must be time for my husband to put the lights on the Christmas tree, because it is the most depressing music imaginable. Every year since I've known him, he plays the entire Messiah while he hangs the lights. I like good music as much as the next person, I just don't find the Messiah to be all that, well, Christmassy. All that talk about spittle and being acquainted with grief makes me need a good rousing chorus of "Grandma Got Run Over By a Reindeer."

Then I think about all of the years of hearing the Messiah with Michael. Our first year, when we went as friends, because I was engaged to someone else. We ran into an ex-girlfriend of his, and I was, to be modest, looking fabulous, 5' 10", 133 pounds, while she, sadly, had signed up with the Date-A-Troll dating service at the time so her escort was not quite, well, human, and she wasn't looking so well either. She tried to make up for it with a silvery laugh, which would have worked had it not turned into one of those last minute snorts. I think it was the best Christmas gift Michael ever received in his whole life until we had kids.

I laugh for a minute about the "perspective lesson" from our first Christmas together. We decided to get a "tabletop" tree for our little apartment. I was picturing something exactly like the one Linus buys in that Charlie Brown Christmas special. Michael brought home a six foot tree. Every year since he has bought a "small tree," which means eight feet.

They were lean years and we were giving each other gift certificates for free things that year. I gave Michael a Football gift certificate, which promised that he could watch an entire game and I would be totally silent. No snappy comments, no observations about those padded pants, nothing about Violence in Society. I could only say these words: "Can I Get You Anything, Darling?" Michael saved that certificate for ten years and presented it to me the day the Packers played the Patriots in the Super Bowl. The man can't find the phone bill from yesterday, but that damn certificate from ten years and three houses ago he finds in 30 seconds. I nearly broke my own jaw keeping that promise.

Fast forward a few years, when EJ is a few months from being born and she seems to respond to the music. She is kicking and kicking away to "He Shall Feed His Flock," a piece which even I love. The concert hall is a little cold and I am as close to Michael as I can get without being entitled to just one ticket price. I tuck his hand on my tummy under mine as we listen and I see tears in his eyes. Admittedly, the man is a blubber head, but I didn't know that yet, because it was having babies that made him that way.

Time goes by, the kids are little. Our Christmas tradition becomes the gospel music Black Nativity or the Nutcracker, or sometimes both. But every year on a Sunday afternoon I still hear those first notes float upstairs.

I look at the clock and realize that an hour has gone by while I've been sitting here daydreaming about Christmases, some so joyous they made me cry, some so painful they did the same. I'm struck by how on each Christmas I wouldn't know what the next one would bring, and that never bothered me before, so maybe it shouldn't now.

I see my reflection in the TV again. The lines are gone. I look awake.

You already know that the contents of your thoughts have a profound effect on your personality. Whatever you spend most of your time thinking about: that's who you are. Awful, isn't it? But try catching a glimpse of your reflection from time to time and you'll know it's true. For me, the Christmas reverie changed my face so much in so short a time that I was convinced.

So I decided that the less I think about cancer, the better. I'm not entirely successful at this, but as I continue to become forgetful I expect that this will become easier and easier. Someday I'll look in my calendar and wonder why I've scheduled a follow-up appointment with an oncologist.

Before you assume that romantic memories alone taught me the lesson of filling my mind with other thoughts besides cancer, please remember that there was chocolate involved.

It's not *all* positive thinking, you know.

SHORTER FUSES

Many people notice changes in their personalities after cancer, which all in all is good. For me, though, I find that I have a lower tolerance for two things, and I'm guessing that you'll find the same thing.

The first is wasting any time at all. I can't stand doing anything that feels like an unnecessary use of time, such as going to long meetings or drying dishes.

The second is complaining. After you've had cancer, you don't spend a whole lot of time complaining about everyday life, and you don't want to listen to anyone else do it either. I used to complain all the time and was happy to listen to other people. Now I want to wear a sign that says "No whining." On a bad day, I just want it to say "Oh, shut up." This feeling hasn't gone away yet and I haven't figured out how to tell someone that a bad condo association meeting is not a tragedy, nor is the price of the ferry to a summer house, and could we please talk about something else.

This makes me realize that cancer may have changed me but it did not make me any nicer.

ODDS – AND ENDS

Remember earlier in the book the part about doctors being trained to have those scientific minds? There is one question you can ask them that will get them touching wood, rubbing rabbit's feet and walking home backwards like the rest of us. Just ask, "How long do I have?"

The only possible answer our doctors could give to this "How long" question is "How should I know?" But we ask them anyway, don't we? Even if they could know, they don't want to tell you. They think that you will feel obliged to die, or maybe that your HMO will just make you go at the appointed hour. Or, if they are wrong and you live forever, they will just never hear the end of it.

For most of us with cancer, who are very, very unlikely to die from it, this question shouldn't come up. But still, if you're like me there will be some dark moment in the middle of the night, when you can't sleep, when you've decided that depression would be a good use of your time, and the only ice cream left in the house is made from soy milk and carob. You decide you want to know just how bad this situation is. And so, even though nobody thinks it's a good idea, you might just go and look up the odds of surviving your stage of cancer for yourself.

Before you go making any plans, like spending all of your retirement money on chocolate and cigarettes just because you think your number is low, take a look at how these odds are decided on.

Let's say you just found out that the odds of surviving your stage are 50 percent.

Five years ago, cancer statistics people took a group of people at your present stage of cancer. Today, five years later, they count how many are alive, and they find 50 percent of them are.

That's how they get your odds. You see? These are not your chances of survival, these are old news numbers about *somebody else's* cancer. So the odds are not based on anything to do with you, your body, your cancer, or your individual chances. And they don't count any new advances that have come along in the past five years.

Also, while they only count the people who actually died of cancer, they include *everybody*. Some of these people were not as healthy as you are, did not go for treatment as you will, or were treated by someone whose medical degree came with free miles.

Still worried? Be sure to read the Stephen Jay Gould article listed in the Cancer Research Plan.

Now you have a choice, because how you use your odds number is, as always, up to you. Does a low number motivate you to fight? Does it make you want to heal with more effort? Then go ahead, tell the whole world you haven't got a chance, if it helps you.

Or are you a person who buys lottery tickets? You are obviously an optimist when it comes to low probability. Mathematicians have discovered that lottery ticket odds are the lowest possible number greater than zero, yet we still buy them. Low odds can't douse hope, so ignore them. They don't apply to you anyway.

My own choice was based on a finely honed understanding of statistics. My chances of living are either 100 percent or 0 percent, since there is no such thing as kind of dead. Since anyone's chances of living forever are always 0, that cancels out the 0 chance, using algebra, in which zero stands for n, which stands for nun, which is who taught me algebra just after turning 150 years old herself. Since the zero cancels, my odds of surviving are 100 percent.

It works for me and I made the honor roll that quarter without actually getting a single correct answer.

HOW CAN MY DOCTOR LIVE WITHOUT ME?

Medical care is another big piece of the transition. During the year of cancer treatment, you live in an incredible medical cocoon. A doctor or nurse will jump to take care of every little thing that happens. Temperature up a tad? Feeling a little tired? Have a cold sore? Feeling a little pain? All of those things that normal doctors laugh at when they get off the phone?

"Please give that Spencer woman some sugar pills to get her to stop calling," your regular doctor says, and the evil nurses laugh and twirl their mustaches.

You can be thankful that oncology is not run by them or by dentists. You know the Latin on the diploma in your dentist's office? It means: "No pain relief for absolutely anyone since 1352." (Note to my dentist: Ha-ha-ha, just kidding, you kind, handsome and painkilling guy.)

Anyway, oncologists are a hypochondriac's dream come true. Whatever tiny little thing happens, they get paged. No sugar pills for you now – they're going to roll out that secret cabinet with all the real medicine in it that you never got to have before. Nausea? Not anymore, my friend. Cold sore? Not for you, our most special patient. Pain? A thing of the past, ma Cherie. You'll think they are Dr. Kildare and that Medicine Woman rolled together (except that this is against hospital policy).

Yes, I know there are good reasons why oncologists treat all these things with such special care. But you're still going to feel that they have taken you to the Special Reserve Private Drug Cellar. And you never, ever want to go back to sugar pills after that.

But then ... it's over. Treatment's done. You'll go for periodic check-ups now. They'll give you a schedule of how often you're going to come back. You won't exactly be there every day anymore.

Then the unthinkable happens: you run into your oncologist's assistant on the street and he doesn't recognize you. Of course, if you ran into your faculty advisor, the same thing could happen. Your obstetrician? Forget it. She wouldn't recognize you even if you were still inside out.

The last day of treatment feels just like the day when your pediatrician, after seeing your darling infant like clockwork for every little check-up, says to you: "See you in a year."

Yikes.

This transition after cancer treatment is like all of those things except scarier. The future yawns ahead a bit and life is supposed to be getting back to normal, except that you can't seem to feel normal. You are beginning to suspect that your doctor is giving you sugar pills again, and you sure miss calling in and getting emergency help for your cold sore.

You expect to be relieved that you won't have all those appointments anymore. But while you had those appointments, there was a feeling of safety. What could possibly go wrong, you think, when I am with these doctors and nurses all the time? *They'll keep anything from happening to me.* You also had the "comfort" of chemotherapy or radiation, so you could feel that something was busy getting rid of those cancer cells. Now that the cat is gone, you picture all those mice coming out from behind the walls.

As I write this I am painfully aware of how stupid it sounds, but I decided at the beginning that this was going to be honest even if that would make it embarrassing. It reminds me of being with a cowboy who tried to teach me how to rope cattle, except I think we were using a barrel, because they don't move as quickly and are only slightly smarter than cows. Anyway, I wasn't doing very well. I had not roped the target once. The cowboy said "I admire you."

I stopped in my tracks, thrilled. Obviously something in my arm, or maybe my wrist, had the Old West in it after all. "Why do you admire me?" I asked, glinting into the sun.

"You could stay out here missing that barrel all day, couldn't you? *You just don't care what anybody thinks.*"

Anyway, I hope that my lack of shame will be your gain. I felt very lucky to be prepared for this post-treatment challenge before it happened. It made me feel more confident that I could live well when treatment ended. I might still have the feelings that I kept hearing about, but at least I would understand them.

For me, that's half the problem, so at least that half was under control. I could approach the end with relief instead of fear, just because I understood the cause. I hope that also works for you.

Of course, you'll continue to see these doctors forever, so it's not total abandonment. I'm just a total break kind of a girl, never one who said "Let's Be Friends," so if I have to let go I'd rather really let go.

Mentally, the day I started taking tamoxifen was hard for me. Sounds crazy, doesn't it, but on that day I felt that oh great, just what I needed, a daily cancer reminder for the next five years. I knew I would get used to it quickly but I still hated the whole idea and the pill sat on my plate, right next to the vitamins, for an hour or so. During this time I read the newspaper, which had a story about tamoxifen. Positive people would take that as a positive sign, but I said that I can't even pick up the f-ing newspaper without thinking about cancer.

Maybe if I suffered from chemo brain I would forget what the pill was for. Maybe if I suffered from chemo brain I would forget what the pill was for. What hill?

That little problem, whatever it was, sure didn't last long.

Back to leaving the medical cocoon. Other than trying to understand why you feel the way you do, I don't have any advice on how to handle this, except to say that you'll get used to it, just as you no longer miss your high school English teacher who loved you so much. (Note to Sister Mary LaScourge: You? No.)

If you are having trouble dealing with post-treatment, by all means seek help or a support group. It can be very comforting to be with people who know what you're feeling and who aren't yet really sick of talking about cancer with you like your friends are.

But if you want to stay connected to the hospital, you'll have to become a volunteer. Hospitals depend on volunteers for many functions, and there are plenty of places for you to help out.

Otherwise, you have to let it go and try to be thankful that you had such great care and seek some help if you need it. You could also try stalking the place, just hanging out there everyday.

P.S. THIS DOESN'T WORK.

"ONLY THE GOOD DIE YOUNG."

My favorite and most comforting prognosis,
and the cancer statistic I most deeply believe.

The Finish Line, For Now And Maybe For Good

THE MUSCLE PAIN FROM PACLITAXEL HAS KICKED IN. I've had my last chemotherapy treatment. I consider myself lucky, because I don't get the numbness that many people get yet, but I do get pretty severe muscle pain. I decide that I'm going to go for my walk anyway. I don't think it's wise to go out having taken pain medication. I figure that endorphins will kick in and cover the pain, so off I go.

I am still middle-aged with bad knees. My muscles are bubble wrap, popping slowly but with every step. Now it's raining, and it's cold. The endorphins don't quite kick in enough and I think I'd better turn back. I pass the contractor on the corner, who cheers me on everyday. Well, actually, he yells me on, like a drill sergeant, me a new recruit.

Maybe today he can see it's not so easy, because he doesn't yell. He smiles, he puts out his hand to high-five me as I go by. His mother has breast cancer and I know he understands why I am out here.

I decide to keep going. Later, when I reach home, I'm walking the Frankenstein walk, legs and arms stiff as boards. I feel as if every muscle will lock if I stop abruptly, so I stretch, but that's not enough. I pick up my free weights and do some lifting. They feel twice the weight they usually do.

I know it's probably not wise, but I lift and lift until every muscle is burning. It takes me forever. My arm is aching from surgery and from a rotator cuff mishap, so in between sets I put a bag of frozen peas on it to give it a break. Again, I know this kind of exertion at this point in treatment is dumb. And if you are ever over at my house for dinner, and I offer you peas, always say no.

I finish the last repetition and head for the hottest and longest shower in human history. I actually feel strong. For the first time, I know that if my cancer ever comes back, I can do this all over again. In the depths of chemo, my darkest fear was that I could never do that, but now I know that I can.

And I think that for today, at least, maybe I'm not a chicken.

LEARNING IS NOT ATTAINED BY CHANCE,
IT MUST BE SOUGHT FOR WITH ARDOR AND DILIGENCE.

—Abigail Adams
Whom I've always admired but am still glad she wasn't my college roommate.

Cancer Information Research Plan

A LITTLE KNOWLEDGE IS A DANGEROUS THING, but not so dangerous as no knowledge at all.

Every patient should have a basic understanding of cancer and its treatment. You want to be well-informed enough to make decisions.

Beyond that depends entirely on you. If your cancer is complicated, your odds aren't great, or if you are uncertain about treatment, then become an expert.

You might also have to become an expert if your cancer is early or small. The number of lawsuits filed against doctors has gone up just a tad, hasn't it, so they don't want to run the chance of missing anything. Even if you tell them that the lump they feel is a clearly visible m & m candy you fell asleep on, there will be a doctor who is ready to wheel out a treatment plan. ("First, we will try removing your left "m." If it melts in my hands, we must remove the &.") There may be debate about using chemotherapy or radiation or not. Talk it over with your doctor, and if you are still uncertain, continue to do research and get other opinions.

Keep in mind that most of us still end up pretty confused, so that your goal is to make the best informed decision you can with as much information as you can. Research is going to help you make a choice, not find the one answer. It might help you to keep that in mind. If you start your quest for information believing that there is a definite answer to a complex question, you'll be looking forever. Cancer is not yet that kind of problem. Someday it will be like strep throat, which used to kill people but is now, if treated, easier than the common cold.

A Soapbox moment: I grew very concerned that a good deal of information is available just online. This can exclude the people who are at greatest risk; poorer women tend to be diagnosed later and die more often. I saw a few "advocacy" fundraising sites that I thought could be happily shut down as soon as the last site visitor has agreed to have an annual mammogram, which was two years ago, and the fundraising could go to early detection in housing projects instead.

Back to research. For a basic understanding, use Level 1. It can be done without Internet access.

To get more detail, more advanced information, and the latest information, move on to Level 2.

THE LEVEL I RESEARCH PLAN: WHAT TO DO IF ALL YOU HAVE IS A PAY PHONE

1. Start by collecting your hospital or doctor's materials on your kind of cancer. Take all of those pamphlets.

2. Call the Cancer Information Service (National Cancer Institute/ National Institutes of Health, the primary government source for information) at 1-800-422-6237. Ask them what they have, they'll send it, and it's all free. I got a package loaded with booklets, a video

and a catalog of other booklets. I called them on Thursday, it arrived on Monday.

3.   Same thing with the American Cancer Society, 1-800-227-2345. One thing I like: they put together a lot of information about your particular type of cancer in one magazine-sized paperback. It's free and it's definitely worth getting.

You can stop right there if you have enough information now. Read something inspirational, like Lance Armstrong's book, and you're done. If your cancer or treatment is complicated or you like knowing more, read on.

You might also want to read more if your cancer is very early. I find that more people are confused about the treatment of early stage cancer for many reasons, partly because you have so many more choices depending on how aggressive you and your doctors want to be.

LEVEL 2 RESEARCH PLAN

Head online, which is the easiest way to learn a little more. You'll be amazed and maybe overwhelmed by the number of sites. By the time you're reading this there are probably a bunch of new web sites that outshine the ones I used. Based on my current experience, I recommend starting at a comprehensive place, like the American Cancer Society (www.cancer.org). For breast cancer, try Komen.org, Imaginis.com, and Rose Kushner's rkbcac.org. Some of the sites, such as susanlovemd.com, include a step-by-step questionnaire that will give you information on what type of treatment to expect. That doesn't count as a second opinion, but you might find it interesting.

Move on to the others as you like – www.Oncolink.com, WebMD.com, the government site of the National Institutes of Health's CancerNet (http://cancernet.nci.nih.gov/ or cancer.gov); Medlineplus.com, Oncologychannel.com, cancereducation.com. One thing I like about cancereducation.com is a feature called "Oncology Week in Review." If you've seen something in the paper about cancer, here's a good place to get a fuller story than you get in your local newspaper. A lot of the site's information is in a video format that my computer wouldn't read, but give it a try.

When you've already learned a lot, try www.asco.org, which is the American Society of Clinical Oncology.

If you are looking for clinical trials, many of the sites in this section will give you information. A good place to start is cancer.gov.

For a description of breast reconstruction, try the American Society of Plastic Surgeons site at plasticsurgery.org. Medem, www.medem.com, has an online medical library that includes some helpful articles on breast surgery/reconstruction. For a useful discussion of the surgery decisions you'll be making, try www.breastcancer.org.

The Breast Cancer section of Feminist Majority is worth a visit (www.feminist.org/other/bc/). Whether you are with them or not politically, they keep a good list of online resources and they evaluate them. So unlike most web sites that just give you a list of links, this one tells you what you'll find there. Great time-saver, plus they cover a wide range of views. Www.Mamm.com also has a comprehensive list of sites, also with descriptions.

There are mailing lists on some of these sites. You sign up, you start getting e-mails. I never did that because my e-mail is already so spammed that I can hardly stand to look at it. The last thing I wanted was to wade through more. You may feel differently.

Many sites focus on education or advocacy, like Lance Armstrong's laf.org. The Avon site, avoncompany.com, and others have a bulletin board if you like those, in which you post public messages and people may respond to them. You can also find a sense of community at the acor.org site (Association of Cancer Online Resources) and susanlovemd.com. Many sites have community sections or even chat rooms and you'll have to do some experimenting to find the right match for you. Try www.gillettecancerconnect.org and Oncochat.org. (Remember to check any information you gather with your doctor.)

You can also try www.cancercare.org for resources on financial help, because cancer can be a challenge if you are already having financial troubles. They list a lot of them and give advice on finding local help. Cancercare.org also gives you resources for finding transportation. If you do not have Internet access, please remember that the hospital where you are being treated will have a resource person to help you. Please ask your doctor or nurse. Try www.y-me.org/ for general information as well as resources for free wigs.

Issues about work? Check out cancerandcareers.org on the Internet. It ranges from information on employee rights to cosmetic help. Cancer Information Service (1-800-422-6237) has a booklet called Facing Forward that covers many employment and insurance issues.

Web addresses change as do services. Ask the hospital for more if you need to.

BOOKS

A note about my book selections. As you know by now, I wanted to spend as little time on cancer as possible, including learning about it. Also, I'm just Stage 3. If I am ever Stage 4, which, God if you are listening, I don't actually want to be, then this list would be different.

There are many good books depending on what you need at the moment. I found it helpful to head for a bookstore, in person or online, a library, or the Learning Center at my hospital and browse to see what fit my need. Here are a few that I liked or loved.

- Lance Armstrong's *It's Not About the Bike* (Berkley). Inspiring, courageous, uplifting.
- *Woman to Woman: A Handbook for Women Newly Diagnosed With Breast Cancer* by Hester Hill Schnipper and Joan Feinberg Berns (Wholecare). It's short and it covers a lot of basics. Has a helpful book list. This is one breast cancer book that I read more than once.
- *Survivor's Guide to Breast Cancer: a Couple's Story of Faith, Hope and Love* by Robert C. Fore, Rorie E. Fore and Nancy W. Dickey

(Smyth & Helwys). In a category of its own.

- An article by Stephen Jay Gould called *The Median Isn't the Message*, from *Bully for Brontosaurus* (W.W. Norton).
- You may already know that *Dr. Susan Love's Breast Book*, (Perseus Publishing) written by a surgeon, is often called the Bible of this field. I confess that I resisted reading it at first, on the belief that no book should be physically bigger than the subject it is about, which this is. I ended up finding it very useful. If you have just read an alternative medicine book that tells you that you don't really need chemotherapy, for example, go here for both sides.
- *Just Get Me Through This! The Practical Guide to Breast Cancer*, by Deborah A. Cohen and Dr. Robert M. Gelfand (Kensington) a very comprehensive practical guide to managing treatment.
- *Bosom Buddies: Lessons and Laughter on Breast Health and Cancer* by Rosie O'Donnell, Tracy Chutorian Semler and Deborah Axelrod (Warner Books).

If you're looking for a deeper view than I wanted, or if cancer has inspired you to change your life in fundamental ways, you'll find many sources of inspiration. Three recommendations to start:

- *Cancer as a Turning Point, A Handbook for People with Cancer, Their Families and Health Professionals*, by Lawrence LeShan (Plume), which my oncologist brother-in-law Rick Rosenberg sent me.
- Margie Levine's *Surviving Cancer: One Woman's Story and Her Inspiring Program for Anyone Facing a Cancer Diagnosis*, (Broadway Books).
- Anything by Herbert Benson, M.D., who runs the Mind Body Medical Institute at 824 Boylston St. Chestnut Hill, MA 02467, (617) 991-0102, www.MBMI.org.

Many people turn to inspirational reading. I received quite a few inspirational books, most of which I couldn't stand, but there were two that I treasured. My friend Roni Pick sent me *For Thou Art with Me*, (Daybreak/Rodale Books) a book which uses the Psalms to give you comfort and encouragement. I was interested because one of the authors (well, besides David) is Rabbi Samuel Chiel. I had heard him speak several times and I couldn't get enough of him. The man doesn't know me from, well, Adam, but I'm a big fan and I love this book.

My niece Christine sent me *Streams in the Desert*, L. B. Cowman, updated by James Reimann, (Zondervan) which gives you a Bible passage and reflection for every day of a year. I looked up my birthdate and it said, from Isaiah 52:12: "you will not leave in haste." Aaaah. This is a book that will carry you through as many days as you wish. If you are a person who likes short stories, you're going to love this approach.

Inspiration is a funny thing; well, actually, it's usually not. I'm not a big reader of books that inspire me by telling me to be inspired. I think you'll find inspiration everywhere around you, and most of it comes from sources that are not at all related to cancer or even illness. I am more moved and inspired by Holocaust survivor Viktor Frankl (*Man's Search for Meaning*) or by soaking in the spirits at Ellis Island. I look at the arrival papers of my great-grandmother, a young widow arriving here with six children and $15. I think about the greatest proof of all that there is always hope in life: people keep having babies under the most unbelievable circumstances.

My point? Seek your own inspiration. My own father has written some pretty inspiring poetry, but I didn't read it during treatment. You may love poetry and find it soothing, I'm just one of those people whose only poetry talent is for limericks. I had two breasts on my chest, till I had my mammography test, that sort of thing. I do like to listen to recordings of Dylan Thomas reading "Do Not Go Gentle Into That Good Night," because while he had a booming deep voice that could be speaking out of a mouth at Mt. Rushmore, the poem is really just a small boy begging "Daddy, please don't die."

However many books you get, please, please, please remember: if you are feeling awful, you are supposed to *call the doctor*. This isn't a cold, so don't try to diagnose yourself, even using a good book.

SUPPORT

Yes, yes, your family and friends are your best support. But many people find that it's comforting to go someplace and talk about cancer or treatment, where everybody there is in the same boat. Your hospital may have good support groups or therapy available, if these would be helpful for you. You may want to start there rather than invest a lot of time and energy in a search for a good match with a therapist, unless you can get some very good referrals.

You're not seeking this support because you're nuts. You're seeking it because it can help you to be stronger, which is going to help you cope, which is going to improve your body. Which reminds me that one of the stupidest research reports I saw was the one in 2002 saying that "support groups have not been proven to reduce the death rate for breast cancer." I have a plan. We go to their research offices and remove anything from their desks that cannot be proven to reduce a death rate. Pain relief. Tampons. Jock itch spray. We keep these things until they know that medicine has many purposes other than reducing a death rate. I give them a day to surrender.

Many people swear by the Wellness Community Centers for all kinds of support. Call 1-888-793-WELL or www.wellness-community.org to see if there is one near you. They offer many free services.

Some of these web sites and phone numbers will give you the option of speaking Spanish. I did not find much printed information in the United States that was available beyond English and Spanish, but there is obviously a great deal of information online in many languages and in printed material in many countries. At www.cancer.org, you can order the Cancer Survival Toolbox which has audio tapes available in English or Spanish; printed copy is provided in Chinese. These items are free as of now. These are useful if someone you know cannot read or prefers to hear information. Imaginis.com has a list of international web sites, including a Canadian site that offers materials in 33 languages.

If you are helping someone who does not speak English, be sure to speak with the hospital interpreter about research. S/he may be more familiar with medical terms than even your best friend is and can be a great person to have on your team.

The first three suggestions in this section are available to everyone. If you don't have a computer, or even a phone, those toll free numbers can be used from a pay phone.

For information on free mammograms and cervical cancer tests (Pap smears), call the Center for Disease Control at 1-888-842-6355. They'll give you a telephone number for your state. If you don't have computer access at home, and you can go to a public library, you may be able to get help using the Internet there.

If that works, you can also try the CDC web site at http://www.cdc.gov/cancer/nbccedp/index.htm. Some public schools will also let you use their computers for access. Your hospital may also have online research facilities for you to use.

If none of this works, be sure to tell your doctor or nurse that you have unanswered questions.

Who Was That Masked Man?

Everyone has asked for the identities of my team. They are:

Oncology	Lowell E. Schnipper, M.D.
Chemotherapy nurse	Holly B. Downing, RN
Oncology Nurse Practitioner	Claire Moroney, RNP
Breast Surgery	Susan Troyan, M.D.
Reconstruction Surgery	Michael Tantillo, M.D.
Radiation Oncology	Abram Recht, M.D.
Radiation Nurse	Donna M. Miller, RN
Primary Care	David Savitz, M.D.
Dentist	James Hirshberg, D.M.D.
Gynecology	Hope A. Ricciotti, M.D.
Therapy	Martha Bagby, M.S.W.
Family therapy advice	George Stavros, PhD.
Hairdressers	Nina Houry and Judi Hartley
Newfoundland hypnotherapy	Ian Simpson, M.D.

Appreciation

APPRECIATION FOR THE CANCER YEAR

My appreciation starts before there is even a book, because there were so many people who got me through this year. This section covers only the treatment period, mainly 2001. There were scores of things that people did that helped me. If you open yourself to it, you're going to be stunned, overwhelmed and healed by kindness. It will carry you across a bridge to the end of treatment and beyond.

My first loves – my husband, Michael, and our kids, EJ and Katherine. My incredible sisters and brothers, Agnes Gootee and her husband Dave, Denise Hughes and her husband Frank, Mike Jerome and her fiancé Herb Williams, Terri Grattan and her husband Bill, Bob Doyle and his wife Monique, Colette Doyle and her partner Laura Gold, who took care of Katherine many times, Frank Doyle and his wife Maureen. My most wonderful in-laws, Mary and Emmet Logan, Cathy and Rick Rosenberg (Rick being an oncologist was a great help), Roy and Lynn Spencer, Sanda and Dave Howland, my world class mother-in-law, Jeanne Spencer, being one of the best people you'll ever meet. My cousin in-law, Dr. Sarah Schaefer, breast surgeon. My dad, George Doyle, and his beloved wife Terry. Uncle Paul and Aunt Gale Schaefer. Uncle Gerry and Aunt Cathy. My wonderful nieces and nephews, especially, not to play favorites or anything, my favorite ones, like those Gootee girls, and Hughes girls, and Jerome boys, and Grattan girls, and Doyle boys and girls.

The most wonderful friends and neighbors in the world. Laura and Steve Loffredo, Laura being the best friend mentioned throughout. Jane Morgenstern and Deb Gaines. Stuart Sadick and James Bryant. Paul McDermott. Kiku Adatto. MaryBeth Elder. My wonderful Aunt Brick, Kathleen McGovern. Judi and John Lauerman. Quita Mullan. Lawrence Baker. Linda and Lenny Delvecchio. Janyce Lee. Denyse and Joe and Erika Bardouille. Hope Ricciotti and Vince Connelly. (Hope is also an obstetrician at Beth Israel and was a visitor at some wonderful moments.) Marie McHugh. Evelynne and Fred Kramer. Elaine Shiang and Fred Li, who inspires me step by step. Barbara and Carl Berke. Ruth Rubin.

And the cooks! Susan Harmon. Kay Harrison. Carol Axelrod and Ed Defranceschi. Jeffrey Vichnick. Elizabeth and Paul Leung. Claire and George Vasios. Susan and Ira Vishner. Alla Urman. Judy Cooper. Carrie King Woodson and Robert Woodson. Suzanne Salamon. Anne Hyde. Katherine Lapuh. Jay Sugarman. Judy Botsford. Barbara Hedges. Cheryl Baressi. Judy Katz and Grant Rhode. Andrea Cohen and Carl Zack. Elana and Bill Givens. Marcia and Donearl Brown.

I found myself to be the luckiest person in the world. Jane Morgenstern, my much-loved friend, also organized the rides and the cooks. Jane is one of those people who builds the community she lives in and is always at the center of positive things. My sister Colette, who managed to view a bat infestation in her house as a sign that I was going to be fine, which you will only understand if you are Chinese. Kiku Adatto, who read to me in the hospital, which I loved. Mary Beth Elder, a fun companion for many trips. Elena Hernandez, who stayed with us after surgery and helped give my kids some normalcy and fun. Aunt Dee-Dee and Uncle Frank Hughes, who received our Katherine as a Boston girl and returned her to us a Southern one. Denyse Bardouille, who arrived with a major wardrobe of bright, happy head scarves.

People like Paul McDermott, Ann Morris, Kathy McCarthy, Roni Pick and Randy Parker, who would just call to say hello. Alan Leventhal's kindness over many years is incredible, but when Fred Seigel and Alan gave me a project to do at the time when I was just ready and anxious to work, it was over the top. Fred brought me back to do more projects at Beacon, which is where I grew up, and so life could feel normal again. You can imagine that I am very grateful for that.

And people who played a special part at each stage: Martha Bagby. George Stavros. Father Wilfrid Dufault. Ruth Rubin. Susan Vishner. Tim Heffernan. Mark Colling. Marcos Santos. Lindy O'Connell. Annette Horwath, Chaim Horwath, Sherry Leventhal, Donna Seigel. Paula Sidman, Ed Sidman, Donna Leventhal, Mark Leventhal, Lionel Fortin, Judi Fortin, Doug Mitchell, Christine Welch, Henry Irwig, Tom Ragno, Erin O'Boyle, Rob Perriello, Mary Perriello, Frances Flaherty, Bill Bonn, Ruben Ceballos. Marty Sleeper. David Summergrad. Devra Lasden. Don Lasden. Vivien Cohen. Anne Wunderli. Stephen Knott. Eileen McGee. Judi Hartley, who shaved my head so memorably. Muriel Leventhal, who doesn't have to do anything but speak to make you remember that you have too much to do to sit around whining, and Norman Leventhal, who is like a son to me and who paid me an unforgettable visit. Nina Houry, who discovered that I am really a blonde.

At the Beth Israel Deaconess Medical Center, I was amazed by the level of patient care. I grew up in a small city, where we not only knew our wonderful doctor, Frank Dufault, but his brothers and kids, too (see Uncle Wilfrid, above). I expected a major hospital like the BID to be impersonal. Instead, it was caring and incredible. And they didn't even know I was going to write a book about it, since I didn't know either. Special thanks to Patricia Black, Michelle Boyd, Thérèse Collins, Rachael Conroy, Karen Dawson, Moh Diallo, Holly Dowling, Suzanne Evaristo, Jennifer Forgione, Abdirahman Hersi, Judi Hirshfield-Bartek, Karen Jenks, Melissa Johnson, Paul and Barbara Levy, Nancy Littlehale, Susan Lubars, Dr. Ronald Marcus,

Bob and Judith Melzer, Donna Miller, Debbie Morales, Claire Moroney, Martin Perry, Ingrid Pitta, Dr. Abram Recht, Radiation; Dr. Hope Ricciotti, my neighbor; Dr. David Savitz, Primary Care; Dr. Lowell Schnipper, Oncologist; Latonya Sims, Dr. Michael Tantillo, Plastic/Reconstruction Surgeon; Dr. Susan Troyan, Surgeon.

In Newfoundland, Dr. Ian Simpson treated me for hot flashes with warmth, humor and hypnosis. Sheila Simpson and Rebecca and Tess English made me feel so welcomed and at home.

When I needed home care after surgery, the nurses were terrific. Kathy Feuerbach and Cathy Davis were my regulars. They personify the nursing profession for me and I'll always be grateful to them.

My chemo buddies were my teenager Elise, whose interest in going moved me deeply, and who even waited on me throughout; (Katherine was too young to go, but helped in so many other ways, especially through her humor and good cheer); my best friend since college, Laura Loffredo, who made me laugh, beat me at word games and relentlessly reminded me to get better; Stuart Sadick, my best friend from first grade, who made me laugh until I had tears streaming down my face and a nurse came in to make sure I was okay; my sisters, Terri Grattan and Colette Doyle, and brothers Bob and Frank Doyle, who gave me one of the best days of my life.

APPRECIATION FOR THE BOOK

I am so grateful to everyone who made this book possible. Michael, as always. Laura Loffredo, who is a better writer and is funnier and who could and does take credit for quite a few of the funnier moments and who wrote this thank you herself. My wonderful friends Jane Morgenstern and Deb Gaines, who were the first to make me believe it was good to laugh about this, not to mention Jane listening to every detail a dozen times. Kiku Adatto, who dragged me through the beginning, the middle and the end. Roni Pick and Paul McDermott, who seemed not to give up on this for even a second when I did. Bill Bonn, Joe Breiteneicher, Randy Parker, Terri Grattan, Colette Doyle and

Laura Gold, Lisa Gold and Karen James, Mike Jerome, Clara Gootee, Denise Hughes and Maegan Guven, who all made me feel it was worth doing.

And the people whose comments came at a crucial moment: My dad, George Doyle. Carol Axelrod, Barbara Hedges, Sonia Irwig, Carl Berke, Evelynne Kramer, Rochelle Cohen, Charlene Higonenq. Marie McHugh, Jan Hinkley, Hope Ricciotti and Vince Connelly. Elena Hernandez. Kara McDermott. Douglas McDermott. Peter Karoff. Ellen Remmer. Jane Maddox. Leslie Pine. Amy Zell Ellsworth. Sally Jackson. Barbara Abramoff Levy. Judy Katz. Eric Buch. Linda Myers. Terri Cohen. Ruth Knott. Mary Motte. Ellen Depelteau. Bernie Margolis, who told me to prove my claim that there is always hope, and get the book done. Sue Troyan, who provided updated information when I hadn't even realized I needed some! And there were two special new people in our lives, Marcela and Juan Uribe.

I was a lucky young woman in college because Angela Dorenkamp was my writing professor. I took her class to avoid taking any literature require-ments, since studying a book pretty much made me never want to read it. Entering Angela's world was dazzling. She is a funny, expansive thinker.

We had to keep a journal every day of personal observations and expe-riences. Being a shallow person, I hated that. "Looked in the mirror, noticed I am really pretty," that was about it for my daily entry. Angela told me to write instead about the two years I had just spent in Hong Kong, little entry by little entry. She knew that I would never be a thoughtful author able to spin chapters out of actual emotions, unlike her favorite student, Laura "To the Lighthouse" Loffredo.

Twenty-five years later, Angela has had a stroke and can't speak. I gave Angela an early manuscript of this book and visited her soon after. I was ter-rified waiting to see what she thought.

I cried my head off, because she managed, with no words at all, to tell me that she liked it. She hugged me, pointed to parts that she liked, and smiled over and over. Thank you, Angela.

I pray a special prayer for Angela now that when she arrives at the pearly gates she will be assigned her very own table, Algonquin style, where she can host the writers and thinkers of her choice from throughout time.

I happen to know that the first philosopher she will pick will be Paul Newman.

Then, enter Paul Levy, President and Chief Executive Officer of Beth Israel Deaconess Medical Center, whose idea it was to publish this by the hospital. Paul is one of those people who are always turning around impossible situations, except that he doesn't end up hated by everyone he turned around. He has an extraordinary mind, meaning that he liked my book. Paul then introduced me to Kris Laping, Senior Vice President of Development, who made it happen and brought so much encouragement and enthusiasm to it, and Larry and Gloria Abramoff, founders of Chandler House Press, who got it done and gave me so much fun along the way. If I were nuts, I would wish I had another disease to write about, because this team is so great, and I thank them from the heart.

BACK TO HANK AARON FOR THE LAST WORD

LAST YEAR, I WAS SORT OF A KID AND I WAS A LITTLE SCARED.
I AIN'T SCARED ANY MORE.

Notebook

PLANNING

Schedule of treatment:

_____

_____

_____

Concerns about daily life:

_____

_____

_____

_____

_____

How I will address those:

_____

_____

_____

_____

HOMEWORK ON HEROES

Heroes I know about:

_____

_____

_____

_____

_____

_____

_____

_____

_____

_____

_____

_____

_____

_____

_____

How they became heroes:

_____

_____

_____

_____

_____

_____

_____

_____

_____

_____

YOU ARE WHAT YOU THINK ABOUT

What are the most important parts of my life?

_____
_____
_____
_____
_____
_____
_____
_____
_____
_____

What reminds me that life is worth living?

_____
_____
_____
_____
_____
_____
_____
_____
_____
_____

Look around: something I've seen that inspires courage:

_____

_____

_____

_____

_____

_____

_____

_____

_____

_____

_____

_____

_____

_____

_____

_____

_____

_____

_____

_____

_____

_____

_____

_____

_____

_____

_____

_____

_____

_____

YOU CAN DO A THING OR TWO

Times when I've used my courage muscle:

_____

_____

_____

_____

_____

_____

_____

_____

_____

_____

_____

_____

_____

_____

_____

My overall goals for most days:

_____

_____

_____

_____

_____

_____

REVIEW

How are things going?

_____

_____

_____

_____

_____

_____

_____

_____

_____

_____

_____

_____

What do I want to change?

_____

_____

_____

_____

_____

_____

_____

_____

_____

_____

LOOK WITHIN

My Strengths:

_____

_____

_____

_____

_____

_____

_____

_____

_____

_____

_____

_____

_____

_____

_____

_____

_____

_____

_____

_____

_____

_____

_____

_____

_____

A Few things I'm going to try:

_____

_____

_____

_____

_____

_____

_____

_____

_____

_____

_____

_____

_____

_____

_____

_____

_____

_____

_____

_____

_____

_____

_____

_____

_____

NUMBERS TO KEEP IN ONE PLACE

ONCOLOGIST

Number   Emergency Number

Nurse   Number

CHEMOTHERAPY NURSE

Number

GENERAL DOCTOR

Number

PHARMACIST

Number   24-hour pharmacy number

BREAST SURGEON

Number   Emergency Number

RECONSTRUCTION SURGEON

Number   Emergency Number

RADIATION ONCOLOGIST

Number   Emergency Number

PHYSICAL THERAPIST

Number   Emergency Number

INSURANCE COMPANY

Insurance Plan Number   Insurance Phone Number

Representative's Name and Number

FAMILY AND BEST FRIENDS

_____

_____

_____

_____

_____

_____

_____

_____

_____

_____

_____

Other medical names and numbers

_____
_____
_____
_____
_____
_____
_____
_____
_____
_____
_____
_____

Sources I want to check for cancer research

_____
_____
_____
_____
_____
_____
_____
_____
_____
_____
_____
_____

Other Phone Numbers I need (Pizza, Taxis, School)

_____

_____

_____

_____

_____

_____

_____

_____

_____

_____

_____

_____

_____

_____

_____

_____

_____

_____

_____

_____

_____

_____

_____

_____

_____

_____

_____

Notes

Quotations are attributed in the text except for the following references.

Page 14 Reference to *The Little Engine That Could* by Watty Piper, Platt & Munk. Do you remember that the Little Engine is a girl train?

Page 16 Reference to "There are no atheists in the foxholes." William Thomas Cummings, attributed in *The New International Dictionary of Quotations*, E.P. Dutton 1986.

Page 26 "stick to your own kind, one of your own kind," from "A Boy Like That," *West Side Story*, Leonard Bernstein and Stephen Sondheim, United Artists 1961.

Page 34 Refers to Sigmund Freud's *The Future of an Illusion*, W.W. Norton.

Page 39 *It's a Wonderful Life*, Republic Pictures, 1947.

Page 43 The sister-in-law is Mary Spencer Logan.

Page 44 The Simpsons™, 20th Century Fox.

Page 51 Yoda is a character from Star Wars, Lucasfilm.

Page 52 Scooby-Doo and Snagglepuss are Hanna-Barbera cartoon characters.

Page 57, reference to aiming for the moon, "The Greatest Salesman in the World," Og Mandino

Page 59 *Fit or Fat*, Covert Bailey, Houghton Mifflin.

Page 59 *The Crying Game*, U.S. Distributor Miramax Films, 1992.

204 • THE COURAGE MUSCLE

Page 61 "Come a Little Bit Closer" by Jay & the Americans, Capitol.

Page 62 "Mayo Clinic Study Finds Optimistic People Live Longer" February 8, 2000, Mayo Clinic, Rochester, Minnesota.

Page 65 "Love means . . ." from *Love Story*, Paramount, 1970.

Page 69 "crisp apple strudel and cream-colored ponies," from "My Favorite Things," *The Sound of Music*, Richard Rodgers and Oscar Hammerstein, 20th Century Fox 1965.

Page 84 ER on NBC.

Page 89 and elsewhere, reference to Dr. Kildare, the television series on NBC from 1961-1966. "How to Handle a Woman," from *Camelot*, Alan Jay Lerner and Frederick Loewe, Warner Brothers; "Macarthur Park" by Jimmy Webb, from A Tramp Shining, MCA; J.K. Rowling's *Harry Potter and the Sorcerer's Stone*, Warner Brothers, 2001.

Page 90 Bob Costas, sports journalist.

Page 96 Reference is to St. John's Wort.

Page 106 "Damn dirty apes" is spoken by Charlton Heston's character in *Planet of the Apes*, 20th Century Fox 1968.

Page 115 "Black Magic Woman," Carlos Santana, The Best of Santana, Sony 1998."In-A-Gadda-Da-Vida," Iron Butterfly, Rhino Records 1995.

Page 121 "Ground Control to Major Tom" from "Space Oddity" by David Bowie, Virgin Records.

Page 130 "Mary Kate and Ashley Clone Themselves at the Dude Ranch" is of course a made-up name. It doesn't refer to any real video created by the girls or their attorneys, who all no doubt have a good sense of humor about this kind of thing.

Page 132 Dear Abby is written by Abigail Van Buren, who is Jeanne Phillips. Doogie refers to ABC's television series "Doogie Howser, M.D."

Page 133 "The Charge Of The Light Brigade," Alfred, Lord Tennyson.

Page 140 The Jetsons refers to the Hanna–Barbera cartoon.

Page 140 Heloise, creator of Hints from Heloise®.

Page 143 *The Picture of Dorian Grey* by Oscar Wilde.

Page 164 "I Get Around" was written by Brian Wilson.

Page 164-165 "Grandma Got Run Over By a Reindeer," by Randy Brooks, various artists. Handel's *Messiah*, George Frideric Handel. The Nutcracker Ballet, based on a book by E.T.A. Hoffman, Music by Peter Tchaikovsky. Black Nativity by Langston Hughes. Charles M. Schulz's *A Charlie Brown Christmas*.

Page 169 Dr. Quinn, Medicine Woman, The Sullivan Company and CBS. *Wit, a Play* by Margaret Edson, Faber & Faber, also on page 92.

Page 172 Frankenstein created by Mary Shelley, as portrayed by Boris Karloff.

Page 188 *To the Lighthouse* by Virginia Woolf, Harcourt.

References to registered trademarks include MAD™ Magazine, Birkenstock®, Jeopardy! (Sony Pictures), Make a Wish® Foundation, Wal-Mart™, AOL®, Mrs. Fields® Original Cookies, Google™, La-Z-Boy®, Tupperware®, Irish Spring®, Guinness®, Canyon Ranch®, Mr. Clean™, Astroglide®, which brings me to ©Chippendales; M&M® is a registered trademark of Mars, Incorporated. Juan Valdez® is a trademark of the National Federation of Coffee Growers of Colombia. Game Boy is a product of Nintendo®. Tower-of-Terror is a copyright and trademark of the Walt Disney Company.

Drug brand names (with generic names)
Chemotherapy: Adriamycin® (doxorubicin), Cytoxan® (cyclophos-phamide), Taxol® (paclitaxel) Hormonal therapy (Note that Hormonal therapy is definitely not HRT, which is hormone replacement therapy.): Arimidex® (anastrozole), Femara® (letrozole), Lupron Depot® (leuprolide acetate for depot suspension), Nolvadex® (tamoxifen). Others: Bellergal® (belladonna/ergotamine/Phenobarbital, Catapres® (clonidine), Effexor®

(venlafaxine), Livial® (tibolone) (not yet available in US), Megace® (megestrol), Neurontin® (gabapentin), Percocet® (oxycodone/acetamino-phen), Tylenol® (acetaminophen).